THE COURAGEOUS CURE

Understanding Why You Get Sick and Revealing How You Can Heal

DR. ALANA BERG, ND

AXIOM HEALTH
PUBLISHING

Copyright and Disclaimers

ISBN: 978-1-9994041-0-9
Axiom Health Publishing

Cover Design by: Charla Maarschalk
Illustrations by: Simon Berg

DISCLAIMERS

There are a few disclaimers I want to make about this book.

1. The first is that this book is not intended to be individual medical advice, but rather used to help you gain greater knowledge and understanding of your health or disease. The information can be used to help you decide which types of doctors, practitioners, healers and/or counsellors you may need in your network to support your individual healing journey. Having been in private practice for over twelve years, I would never presume to understand the intricate complexities of your individual health picture without a proper assessment, and the same applies to this book. As such I, in the roles of both a Naturopathic Doctor and author, take no legal responsibility for your individual health. This is medical information, not advice, and should be treated as such. There are no warranties or guarantees expressed or implied by the medical information provided in this book. You must not rely on the information as a personal alternative to medical advice from your doctor or other professional healthcare providers. You should always be working directly with health care providers on answers to your specific questions and concerns for your health. Any action that you take based upon the information in this book, you do so at your own risk. We (author and all others associated with this book) will not be liable for any losses or damages in connection with the use of this information.

2. There are several patient examples in this book. Names and specific details have been changed to protect their identity, unless I have had written

approval to share their specific stories. So, although these stories are true in their main aspects, the details in some may differ from the actual events. In some cases, details have been combined from a selection of patients to protect identities yet provide a representative example of that type of story.

3. In this book I refer to God or Jesus in relation to the spiritual self that comes to be known in the deeper levels of healing. If this is not your conviction, fear not, for this is not a book about your salvation. The essence I want to portray is that of a connection to a power greater than yourself, that influences you, guides you, and transforms you. It is ultimately represented in the grace and unconditional love for oneself and for others. God is love. You may prefer a name such as The Higher Self, The Universe, Holy Spirit, Intention, Highest Potential, Grace, God Within, Angels, Creator, Vital Force or any other name more meaningful for you. I use God or Jesus in alignment with what makes sense for me, and for the sake of simplicity, do not always expand on other types of spirituality, but you can substitute the words that are more authentic to your own beliefs, whatever they are. This book is not intended to be a debate of the merits of any one type of faith, but rather is intended to foster a deeper understanding of the uniformity of the human experience – regardless of race, ethnicity, religion, sex or any other definition that causes division in our society rather than connection. How you choose to connect to that spiritual identity is your innate right. I will be talking about the commonality of our spiritual being and its connection to our health and healing. So please understand no offense nor specific dogma is implied in my writing, just an exploration of common values through the lens of my own experience.

Dedication

To my beloved husband, Robertson
and my precious girls, Myla and Haylee.

Contents

Acknowledgments

This book has been an accumulation of ten years of unrelenting desire, and finally 2 years of intense action. For those ten years, I felt a divine calling to write, however had a million and one reasons why I couldn't. When I finally decided to step forward into the decision, I thought the hard part was over. Ha! It's been the most challenging yet exhilarating process that I could have ever imagined. I have felt so many emotions from confidence when the words flowed, to guilt at the sacrifice of time, to confusion on how to create this book, to overwhelm once I figured that out, to gratitude when the right people crossed my path at the right time, to disappointment when things didn't always work out, to fear when sometimes they did. I have to say this whole process could not have been possible without the people around me in my life to encourage me when I faltered, remind me of the dream I was following when it was tough, and celebrate with me when I achieved a goal. I couldn't have been more blessed!

I have to thank the Lord my God for being with me every step of the way. For setting a fire in my heart to share with the world my desire to see all people healthy, empowered and thriving! This journey has been a huge walk of faith, and I have seen so many gifts and blessings along the way!

To my family, words can't describe how much I love you!

To my amazing husband, Robertson Fait, I can't thank you enough for your endless love and support. You are my best friend and number one support. In the past two years you have gone above and beyond to give me the time I needed to focus on creating this book. Thank you for sacrificing so much for our family and encouraged me to follow my dreams. I am truly able to be the best version of me, because I have you by my side.

To my beautiful children, Myla and Haylee. You make my world shine each and every day. I am so privileged to be your mother, and I am so thankful for the lessons you teach me each and every day. Thank you for forgoing play dates and story times with me, so that I could write the book. I pray that one day you too will follow your passions in every capacity that you desire.

To my loving parents, Allan and Lois Berg. Thank you for always being there for me. I am incredibly blessed. You have taught me values of determination, tenacity, courage, and integrity; all of which have made this book possible. Even at times when you didn't agree with all of my "big ideas," your love has been unwavering. You have allowed me the gift of spreading my wings onto my own path. Thank you for helping me with a final edit to this book, and always being my biggest fan.

To my talented brother, Simon Berg, thank you for creating the amazing graphics in my book! I know they were often under tight deadlines from a simple scribbled diagram! Thank you for being so flexible and efficient!

To my dearest friend Charla Maarschalk, you have been so instrumental in the creation of this book. I don't know if thank you can really represent my gratitude! Your creative genius astounds me. From the amazing book cover, to the last minute photoshoot, to the desperate web design, to any design for that matter, to the needed emotional support; I am so lucky to have such an amazingly gifted woman as such a kindred friend. Thank you!

To Antonio Jimenez, unbeknownst to us, God had a plan when we met back May 2017. Thank you so much for writing the forward in my book, and for being such an inspirational friend. You are doing God's work.

To the most determined and resourceful woman I know, Jessie Puetz, thank you for taking charge on my book launch celebration, and helping me along the way when I needed a road runner. I'm blessed to have such a caring friend in my life.

Thank you to my good friend Yolanda Dye for giving the push to start this book journey. I really needed that kick! Thank you to Chantel Adams for helping me find my story to share. Thank you to Joanna Bell for my book editing. Thank you to Krista Goncalves for helping sort this whole process out, yikes I needed a lot of help! Thank you to Jennifer Sparks for formatting the book, and bringing it to publication. Thank you to my videographer, David Hughes marketing master Mark Tompkins, and website designer Chris Stephens.

Thank you to my good friends and family: Kellie, Krisstael, Cheryl, Janel, Robyn, Rachel, and Shannon for being my sounding board: for sometimes just listening, for sometimes giving advice, and for sometimes just bringing the wine.

Thank you to my friends and colleagues Audrey Wolter, Diego Navarro, Josep Soler, Daniella Demarche, Greg Hofmann, Trevor Hoffman, Ara Elmajian, Rick Klippert, Hugh Thompson, Grant Pagdin, and Esther Simmons Foot for years of support, mentoring, collaboration and the gifts that you bring to the world.

I hope you enjoy reading this book as much I did writing it. There was a huge process of self-discovery in putting this out into the world. I pray that it can also launch you into your own journey of self-discovery!

Foreword

DR. ANTONIO JIMENEZ, M.D., N.D., C.N.C.

During my travels around the globe, I have had the opportunity to meet many noted physicians whose views I have integrated into my understanding of the human disease and healing experience. Among them, every now and then, I have encountered individuals who demonstrate a sense of connection with their profession that transcends that which a diligent acquisition of knowledge alone can provide. One such rare individual is Dr. Alana Berg, who I have had the privilege of interacting with at several naturopathic doctor conferences, and who I consider an esteemed colleague and friend. Physicians like her share a unique sense of commitment towards their patients, seeking healing unfettered by the self-imposed limitations of viewing disease through the erroneous lens of symptoms alone.

Even though our individual experiences and pivotal moments may have been radically different, Dr. Berg has traversed a journey of self-discovery that I find very relatable. Within her story you will find her "why," the seed to who she has become – the "magic sauce" that gives special meaning to her life's work. By finding the courageous cure within her, she has committed herself to encourage others to find it within themselves. In that sense of caring responsibility, I find the essence of what makes a true healer.

Why do I consider this book a must-read? Of course, the book is dotted with freely shared pearls of medical knowledge, waiting to be uncovered by you – which should be a good enough reason, regardless of your existing medical belief system. However, Dr. Berg also does not shy from treading the fine line between fact and philosophy, bringing astonishing clarity to incredibly abstruse ideas. Even as I read this book, I was elated to find some of my previously nebulous thoughts translated into words that help me give them expression. I can guarantee that reading this book will give you a surprising insight into the workings of your own body, as long as you keep an open mind. You will finally understand that you were designed to be a supremely empowered being, capable of finding your own path to healing.

If you have cancer or another serious chronic disease, I believe this book has been written for you more than anyone else. Dr. Berg will inspire you to look for solutions to your malady in places that you may least expect. When conventional medicine says there is no other way, Dr. Berg will show you the path to discover your own courageous cure.

Dr. Berg, we thank you for this treasure trove – many blessings for your continued good work and discovery!

By Dr. Antonio Jimenez, M.D., N.D., C.N.C.
Founder and Chief Medical Officer
Hope4Cancer Treatment Centers

Introduction

This book has been a concept of mine for over ten years, but for many reasons (or shall I say excuses), I never got around to writing it. I would have said "I didn't have time", or "I didn't need to write it" – maybe a sentiment you can also relate to about a goal you have had in your life. Yet, if I'm truthful, I put it off more out of the fear of criticism or rejection – and maybe even of success.

However, the idea to write this book became a lot more personal to me a few years ago, with the birth of my first daughter. This life-changing event fuelled me to share my own personal experience, and how it related to my basic desire to empower you in your health journey. The concepts I outline here in the book have been discovered and developed throughout my personal journey, my many years of clinical experience, and my constant pursuit of learning from great minds in my field. I want nothing more than for you to take control of your health, and in turn take back your life. I pray that's exactly what this book can do for you.

As a Naturopathic Doctor, and a self-expected high achiever my whole life, I assumed when it came to this whole birthing thing, I'd have it mastered. Women have been doing it since the dawn of man. I knew my anatomy and physiology inside and out. I knew exactly what that process was…textbook. Looking back, I probably could have used a little bit of healthy curiosity and caution about how that might apply specifically to me, but even the pain didn't scare me. I had a plan after all. I didn't make it through university and naturopathic medical school without a very clear plan.

However, what I experienced was a very different story from what I had read. My labour likely started like many labour stories, slow and steady – the only problem was, I wasn't dilating. As the contractions got closer, my pain increased, along with my expectation that my beautiful baby was going to be with us shortly. But after eighteen hours, and some pretty intense contractions every minute, I was only 2.5 centimetres dilated. My midwife noted, "There is nothing like a well-timed epidural," to encourage me to manage the pain. Thinking about my birth plan, that was the last thing I wanted to hear, but in terms of the pain intensity – it was the only thing I wanted to hear. Unfortunately, I wasn't a great candidate for a "walking" epidural. It didn't change the pain level significantly, nor did it slow down or reduce the intensity of my contractions.

I went another ten hours before I finally made it to 5 cm – exhausted and starving, but determined to have my baby naturally. Transition, which is the period of time where most women will have the most intense contractions and pain while the cervix finishes dilating to 10 cm, lasted for a total of four more hours. In that process, exhausted and depleted, I hit a breaking point. I'm not sure I was coherent enough to have a rational thought about it, but I can remember feeling like I was detached from my body, like I was watching myself. Trauma happens when you go beyond the point where you can cope. Although I didn't know it at the time, that breaking point was the moment that triggered post-traumatic stress and set a course for a series of health issues down the road.

I eventually did manage to muster the last bit of strength I had to push my beautiful baby out and into the world – nearly thirty-four hours after labour began – but the state I was in at that point was very different than what I had expected. Being a doctor, I "should have" recognized I had PTSD (Post-Traumatic Stress Disorder), but at the time, I just knew the birth was unbelievably difficult, and I could never imagine doing that again. I went home the next day with my precious baby girl, but it was hard and I struggled. It took me three weeks to leave my house, six weeks to figure out how to nurse without being in pain, and eight weeks to physically heal from the birth (and literally, to urinate without pain), but I was determined – I knew what I should be doing, therefore I would do it. I would get up and move on.

At about three months' postpartum, I woke up one morning with my daughter lying beside me, and my right arm was completely numb. I thought I must have pinched a nerve, sleeping in an awkward position, and figured it would go away. So I pushed on. Being a self-employed doctor and our family's income generator, I had only allowed myself four months of maternity leave before I decided I had to go back to work. I felt I *had* to keep going. My husband stayed home, and I was balancing work and being a new mom. I often felt like a milk factory – constantly pumping in between patient visits and on lunch breaks. It was so important to me to give my daughter the best start possible, that I was oblivious to the consequences on my own health.

I was like a zombie going through the motions of early mommy-hood. I was pushing through, and all along continued to have this numb arm. I connected with my resources and colleagues. I tried massage, chiropractic care, injections, physiotherapy and acupuncture, to no avail. I finally decided I needed more information, and I went to get a private MRI done, so I knew what was going on.

I thought it would likely be a pinched nerve in my arm, brachial plexus, or neck, so I felt pretty confident that this annoying numb arm would have a quick and easy recovery. Only the report came back showing demyelination in my neck and a recommendation to get a brain scan as well. Demyelination is when the myelin sheath that wraps around the nerve is damaged thereby effecting the conduction of a nerve. I went in for a brain scan, which also showed demyelination in the brain. Shocking! I saw two different neurologists who both believed that I had Multiple Sclerosis (MS), which the reports had alluded to. This left me feeling stunned, as I'm sure many of you can relate to when you hear unwanted, startling news.

It's like the illusion of the past year all came crashing down. I was exhausted, but I just knew in my heart that MS was not my story. I was determined to create a different reality. I walked out of their offices telling them I wasn't interested in prescription drugs, and knowing the only way they'd see me again was if I came back to tell them "I'm cured!"

I knew when I really looked at my situation, my symptoms were not some random areas of the brain with inflammation and damage with unknown origin, but that there was a bigger message. So I did some soul searching, and I started a journey of transformational change.

I worked for two years on that process of healing, determined that MS wasn't going to be my story. I utilized all the tools, resources and knowledge that I had available, all of which I will be sharing with you in this book!

I immediately changed my diet to gluten free, sought out healers to work with, and started supporting my adrenal health and hormone balance. I reached out to my network of trusted practitioners (a cranial sacral therapist, acupuncturist, BodyTalk practitioners, counsellors, massage therapists, chiropractors and fellow NDs) and I intuitively went to each of them when I felt they would assist in my healing journey. I treated my episiotomy scar with neural therapy to clear my body's energetic hold on the trauma (which we will discuss later in this book). I also started to pray, because I believe God brings people into our lives that have the gifts needed to help us heal, as well as bringing us miracles. I prayed for a miracle.

When I got to the place where I was finally looking deeply inside, rather than outside for healing, things really shifted. When I went inwards, and asked the question why – my intuitive heart knew the truth. *I was not letting myself heal from the trauma of my daughter's birth.* I knew that something had changed in me at that moment, and I hadn't felt like myself ever since.

I had revelations about my coping process and what I needed to let go of. I was also coming up to a place in my life where I actually had a desire to have more children. It had been out of the question up to that point, so I knew it was a hurdle I would have to overcome. I began to talk about my experience for what it was, and felt a release of all the emotions I had kept stuffed up inside: the fear, the failure, the shame, the pain. I had finally realized I had to forgive myself and accept what had happened, in order to let it go.

Forgive what? Well, I thought that intellectually I should've known what labour was like; I had anticipated the birth would follow a predictable path. When my experience, however, turned out to be quite different from what I expected, it left me feeling defeated. I realized I needed to forgive myself for not knowing it all, for being human, for being vulnerable and for being imperfect. I held onto such a strong contradiction inside between what I *expected* of myself versus what I *experienced* that I had literally stopped my body from feeling. I numbed myself!

Within this process I finally found a neurologist that was willing to work *with* me, accepting my stance on the diagnosis and treatment. He suggested we have a repeat MRI, as it would be the only definitive way to determine if I did in fact have MS – since MS is a progressive disorder, there would be indications of new lesions by that time. I hadn't had any new symptoms since the first onset, and knew in my heart I was ok, but it still terrified me to go. The perceptions of the world around us, despite what we know intuitively, have the potential to shake us all to the core.

I continued to pray, had my MRI before Christmas, and then left on a wonderful trip with my family for the holiday season. I was finally starting to feel like myself, and my daughter was nearly two and a half years old! Shortly after arriving home, I found out I was pregnant. I was both excited, because I knew I was in a better place, and scared, because things with my health were still unknown.

Then finally, it was time to get my results. I went to my appointment and the neurologist said that he didn't know what happened – there were no new lesions, and even evidence of healing in previously abnormal areas... It was my miracle!

I went on to have another beautiful healthy little girl, all natural labour and in only six hours from start to finish. It was hard, as all labours are, but I was in a completely different headspace than the first time. I also never had, and still don't have, any reoccurrence of numbness or symptoms. As far as the conventional health system and my insurance companies are concerned, I have and always will have the diagnosis of MS, but I know personally that MS is not my story.

This is my miracle in my life, and it is part of why I do what I do. It encourages me to want to share my message with the world. The understanding of my own health story has shifted how I practice medicine, and how I approach healing entirely. My goal for this book is to inspire you to understand that you too can take hold of your own health journey and change the story that you have been sold.

The current dominant medical model in our modern culture has its limits, and is not designed to instill self-awareness and self-empowerment. It's a reactive medicine, not a proactive one. So, we do not have to be victims of our reality; we can actually create it. When we understand the real underlying causes of our illness and imbalances, and heal at those levels, then we can take hold of our future.

I want you to know how and why we can heal ourselves, to understand the depths of what our bodies are trying to tell us, and to discover the inherent knowledge that we all have for healing, if we can just tap into it.

There are layers to our illnesses that involve every aspect of our lives, and I often tell my patients that we are peeling back these layers like an onion as we move through the process of healing. Since we are complex and interconnected, we are required to look at healing through the same lens of complexity and interconnectivity. There is no one magic recipe, one cure-all pill, because we are not all the same. We tend to tune out our body's messages and follow along with what the world is saying we're supposed to do. Instead, we need to tune in to what the body is saying on each level. In my own experience with illness, I had to go through the foundational levels of healing to resolve my symptoms. In this book, you too are going to discover what your root causes of disease are, what levels of healing you need to address, and how you are going to heal yourself.

If you are suffering from any chronic disease like Inflammatory Bowel Disease, Lupus, arthritis, allergies or any other inflammatory or autoimmune disease, this book is for you. If you have cancer and are feeling stuck in how to move forward, this book is for you. If you have been left without support or answers about your health problems, this book is for you. If you are feeling scared of a medical diagnosis you have been given and what sort of future you may hold, this book is for you. If you want to prevent disease and become the best version of yourself, this book is for you. If you just feel stuck and tired, and have no idea what needs to change (but know that something does), this book is for you. If you are feeling broken, hopeless, depressed and alone, this book is for you. If you are feeling like you want to tap into and reveal the uniqueness of you, this book is for you.

You are the courageous cure.

You will need courage to *own* your personal story: to take responsibility for who you are, or what you have become, and to take the reins back, and start to navigate your health journey on your terms.

At times it will be difficult, grueling, exhausting, overwhelming or even frustrating, but with persistence, tenacity, perseverance, grit, devotion and resilience you will overcome. You will find the courage to face your challenges straight on, and in doing so, will transform who you are. You are the creator of your cure.

Part One

There Are Deeper Roots to Illness: Symptoms Are The Messenger

"If someone wishes for good health, one must first ask oneself if he is ready to do away with the reasons for his illness. Only then is it possible to help him."

~ Hippocrates

Root Causes of Disease

When I see patients for the first time, I always begin with explaining my background and training. I relay that my training is similar to a Medical Doctor's, as most people are familiar with this – first going to university for Pre-Medical education and then another extensive four years of medical school. The key difference with the Naturopathic Doctor's training is the *approach* to healing, which changes the type of treatments used. Our focus as NDs is to figure out *why* things are happening, not just *what* is happening, in order to get to the root cause of disease. The roots may have layers, like an onion, depending on how long the symptoms have been there, how severe they are, and how many systems in the body are being affected. We often must clear up one layer, before another one can be revealed. This approach views healing as a process with multiple levels, rather than a single treatment or prescription. The symptoms you experience are your body's method of communication, telling you all that needs to be considered. A sort of way of saying, "Pay attention, we need to deal with this."

I have also had several patients over the years say, "If it was any other symptom, I could deal with it, but this…this I cannot."

And I say, "Exactly! Everything else that did show up didn't get your attention, so now it's just speaking louder." Hence, if all we ever do is focus on that symptom – suppress it, cut it out, burn it off, etc. – we miss the message. And the body will continue to try to get our attention, unfortunately sometimes to the point where it stops us in our tracks. I see this often with skin rashes, like eczema. A steroid cream is often prescribed to "suppress" the rash, so that the symptom goes away. However, the "message" now shows up somewhere else in the body – for example, commonly in the digestive tract with symptoms such as diarrhea, constipation, bloating or cramping. So how do we get a handle on these things sooner? How do we discover the messages earlier on?

For starters, we need to start to pay attention to what's really going on. In order to get to the root of the problem, it is important that we look at the whole picture. We are not robots, we are a holistic system – physical, energetic, emotional, mental and spiritual – intricately designed and connected. We cannot treat one level and not expect it to influence another. We need to start to shift our paradigm awareness on how the body works, all these systems fitting together to make a whole.

So often I tell my patients that when we are bringing the body back into alignment, I don't know at what point the symptoms will shift – right at the beginning of our treatments, near the end, or somewhere in between – but when the symptoms message no longer needs to be relayed, then the symptom no longer needs to present itself.

Now I'm not suggesting that we necessarily avoid symptoms, as they can be very debilitating and even an obstacle to getting into a practitioner's office, but it's important to understand the paradigm shift between *root* focused and *symptom* focused. This understanding will help you realize where you need to start looking for a cause.

In Part 1, I will reveal the biological and environmental factors that are at the root of our diseases, the obstacles which are blocking the body from being its vibrant self. I will lay the groundwork for deciphering what your roots are. Then in Part 2, you will know which levels of healing are required from those root causes.

So let's discuss what the root causes of disease are. Through my years of practice, as well as from the teachings of some pretty amazing leaders in the medical and naturopathic community, I have noted some specific keys that are the main root causes of disease. In looking at these roots, there isn't any disease that we cannot break down into one or several of these root causes. Sometimes the hardest part is knowing where to start first. We then need to determine how many roots we are dealing with, and which the most important priority is.

These are the categories of root causes I will detail in Part 1, to help you understand them fully – as well as what to do about them.

1. Genetics
2. Nutrient deficiencies
3. Toxicity
4. Chronic infections
5. Electromagnetic frequencies
6. Stress and trauma

Most of us don't have just one root, but rather several. The more you understand each root cause, the more that you will be able to determine which ones you need to work on. We are going to dissect each one, and although at times the content may seem heavy, please know in my effort to be thorough I've included a lot of information. I would rather explain each of these with more material than less. While I may touch on some methods that may be used in treatment, I will expand in detail on the healing methods in Part 2. The objective of Part 1 is to get the full understanding of the roots of illness, before we jump into healing in Part 2.

In the next several chapters, my desire is for you to truly comprehend the depths of why we get sick. You are the author of your life and your health, and with this information comes realization and empowerment to make change. This path may seem daunting at times, but please understand that it first starts with a choice - a choice that says, "No, this is *not* me, I *am* choosing a different way." You may come up against skepticism or even disapproval for expanding your knowledge outside of "mainstream" medical conventions, but remember, no other human on this earth has authority over your health and wellbeing. You are its sole director, its author, its interpreter.

There are examples throughout history of people embracing change and rising up against adversity. They are people that instigate innovation with courage, and inspire us to do the same. Sending a man to the moon, inventing the computer, discovering antibiotics – nor the multiple inspiring actions in personal life stories like Mother Teresa's or Gandhi's – are not small feats, and neither is your action to make real, lasting change happen in your life. These were normal people like you and me, with a divine purpose to achieve their goals, no matter the cost. Your cost is embracing change and opening up your mind to the possibility that there is another way, another truth, another life. To be responsible for your life, and accountable for its outcome. To know that your soul's desire is to be the best version of yourself: the healthiest, the most energetic, the most passionate, the most empowered, the most peaceful, the most free, the most alive.

Becoming your optimal vital self requires you to take care of yourself. You are responsible for your actions, beliefs and thoughts. You own your story and your destiny. You have a reason to live! I want nothing more than for you to unlock your internal greatness, and fulfill your individual, unique purpose in this life. When you don't meet your full potential, you deprive someone else of the experience of being with the most authentic, inspiring you. The one and only you. *Believe that you can change your story and in turn change your life*. It's time to remove the shackles of limitations and "be the change you wish to see" (Gandhi).

ONE

Genetics

"Epigenetics doesn't change the genetic code, it changes how that's read. Perfectly normal genes can result in cancer or death. Vice-versa, in the right environment, mutant genes won't be expressed. Genes are equivalent to blueprints; epigenetics is the contractor. They change the assembly, the structure."
~ *Bruce Lipton*[1]

When my mom first started experiencing weakness in her legs and a poor gait, which made her more prone to falls, she resolved to meet a specialist to determine what was going on. She was concerned because her own mother had very similar symptoms that started years before with a confirmed diagnosis of Desmin Storage Myopathy, a rare muscle dystrophy disease. It is a "genetic" disease that doesn't present symptomatically until a person is in their 50s or 60s – and being 54, she knew that there was a possibility. Her mother had been diagnosed in her early 60s, and although she also experienced weakness, really didn't seem to be too physically inhibited until her later years. In her late 70s, she began to require a cane, and then a walker, and finally a help button because of her inability to get up from the floor in case of a fall.

So when the diagnosis of myopathy came for my mother (as well as her sister), she knew things might be hard, but that she would be ok. She watched her mom struggle with mobility later in her life (while also suffering from diabetes and congestive heart failure), but she did continue to walk right up to the end of her life – literally to the moment when her leg bones broke from her own body weight when her leg muscles gave out. My grandmother never came out of the hospital after that fall, and died in her 82nd year. My mom witnessed that experience, and although unpleasant, felt like she had a lot of time before she would come close to the same fate. So, she was surprised when she experienced quicker deterioration – by age 67 she required a cane full time, had to limit her outdoor adventures to only handicap accessible options, and most unfortunately, had to give up on some of her dreams to travel to distant far off places. She has also had several falls from loss of balance and weakness, much like her mother, resulting in injuries, breaks, and concussions. And although she lives to the fullest that she can right now, she inevitably continues to show slight progression of this disease.

Medicine of the past century is a result of the belief that we are a product of our genes. Genes are the unique code embedded within the molecular makeup of each and every cell of your body, and make you who you are. The genes are housed in the nucleus of the cell, which for decades was believed to be the brain of the cell. Many scientists believe that what a cell does or doesn't do is determined by the genes. The belief is that who we are is predetermined in the womb – what diseases we will manifest, what behaviors we will express, and how our physical body will look and respond. The modern medicines we have today are meant to control symptoms, because they are based on the belief that no matter what we do, our genes will determine our future. That the path has already been written based on generations of history.

Now, before I continue, I must say that through this model humans have discovered many lifesaving procedures and medicines that have revolutionized our response to emergency situations. Out of the dawn of the World Wars the discovery of morphine, antibiotics and vaccines not only allowed for much more humane treatment, but also saved lives. Many people with acute injuries and infections that historically would kill them, were now able to survive. The extension of the theory, however, of a single pharmaceutical cure into every aspect of medicine, including chronic disease, is where we have lost momentum. The rates of chronic diseases such as cancer, heart disease, allergies, arthritis and autoimmune diseases are ever increasing, while overall mortality has decreased. So we may be living longer, but are we living well?

What has been realized in the last fifty years, and largely popularized with the help of Dr. Bruce Lipton (among others), is that epigenetics is a much stronger indicator of your overall health and wellness. In the description of epigenetics, our genes are seen as simply a blueprint – instructions, based on generations of environmental exposures, on what the body could do or create when exposed to different environments. In fact, Dr. Lipton found that a cell could even live for a period of time without its genes at all, the part that had previously been thought of as the most important part of the cell. How could that be?

When you build a house with blueprints, they're going to give you instructions on how to build that house. If you take those blueprints away, you could still build that house – but without instructions, your chances of success will be slim. Adapting to environmental changes, such as weather changes for example, would be very hard. So eventually that house will not be very structurally sound, and will likely crumble with exposure to the elements. Like blueprints for a house, your cells need the genes in your nuclei to give them instructions on how to *respond* to the "elements" or environment they're exposed to. The adaptability and survival of each cell depends on it. We even have two different blueprints to pull from, one from our mother and one from our father! We cannot survive without genes, but they are not actually the most important area of the cell.

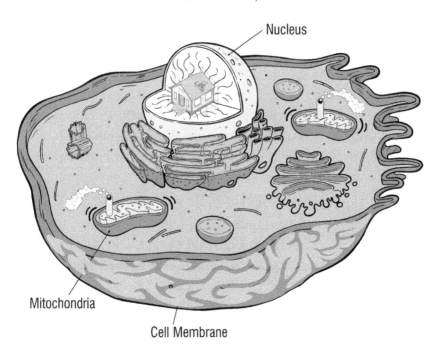

So if the nucleus of genes isn't the dictator of cell function, what is? The cell membrane, whose surface acts as an interchange to the outside world, constantly seeking out and bringing back messages to the nucleus about what is going on and what is needed to be created. It is the "sensor" to anything outside the cell. This feedback helps us to know how to respond to the environment, acting as a "brain" for our cells, so to speak. The cell membrane takes in information about the environment through its receptors – much like our brains take in stimuli through touch, taste, sight, smell or hearing. This membrane "brain" conveys to the cell this environment, and then the nucleus infers which genetic "blueprints" are the most appropriate to build that strong "house" in response.

So, if the genes are the blueprints, and the membrane is the brain, what actually makes those cells do their work? Well, it's actually our second piece of DNA – little microbial DNA called the mitochondria – that produce energy for the cells to function. Think of them as our energy factory: when we breath and eat, the mitochondria create energy for us, using both oxygen and the components of our food that act as the building blocks for that energy. The mitochondria are the energy work horse, and without them, the cell would not survive. We have ten million billion mitochondria in our body, and they produce both energy molecules (40%) and heat (60%). We need those energy molecules, called adenosine triphosphate, or ATP, to be made for every little thing we do: every movement, every breath, every cellular change, every enzymatic reaction, every bit of metabolism. We literally produce seventy kilograms of ATP daily (recycled 1000 times a day), just for use at rest! Everything requires energy. Just as we can't build that house without blueprints and a brain to decipher which blueprint to use, we can't build it without our energy "workers," mitochondria, either.

Damage to any one of those areas – the nucleus, the cell membrane or the mitochondria – by exposure to different negative environments – like toxins, infections, radiation or stress – will all influence the cell function. Even how we feel about something can influence cell function. It can change your DNA (genes), it can change which gene your cell decides to express (membrane), and it can shut down the energy production that the cell needs (mitochondria).

What does this all mean for you? Genes outline how your body is created and how it works. Depending on provisions in the environment, mutations and family genetic patterns could be passed on. When we perform genetic testing, like "23 and me" for example, we're really just seeing a blueprint of what could potentially happen. We should be careful not to use this testing as a "crystal ball" into some predestined future, potentially creating fear of outcomes beyond our control. Rather, we need to look at the results with the perspective that those inherit genetic weaknesses can give clues on how to optimize our milieu to best influence our genes. Through adjustments to diet and lifestyle, as well as providing a good clean environment to live in, we can be enabled to maximize our genetic potential.

So how does this apply to my family? Conventional wisdom would tell you that the health outcomes determined by your genetic pool are the end of the line and there is nothing you can do to stop it. But this is absolutely not true. To the contrary – my grandmother was the first in her family to manifest this genetic disease. What does this mean? Since there were no other ancestors that had any type of muscular dystrophy, it's more than likely there was something in her life that triggered or changed a gene in order to express the disease. What could it be? Possibly the severe rheumatic fever she had at age twelve that kept her hospital bound for five months, or perhaps the chronic stress she was under as a mother of four, living on a farm, in an unhappy marriage. Her home for 95% of her adult life was an old farmhouse on a crop farm – with well water, agricultural sprays, lead paints and lead pipes. She also seemed to have a negative outlook on life that unfortunately left her feeling pessimistic and filled with worry. Any of these elements, or a combination, could have triggered the genes' expression of myopathy. It is also interesting that only my mother and one of her sisters, out of the four sisters in the family, were actually diagnosed with the disease.

As for my mom, well along in her journey to discover wellness, she found out that she had been gluten intolerant – likely for over fifty years as she had suffered chronic bowel issues and constipation for much of her life. My mom also had some of the highest heavy metal loads I have ever tested, and I have tested hundreds of people over the years. She had high levels of lead, likely from the well water on her childhood farm. She also had a mouth full of mercury amalgams that left her riddled with high mercury levels in the body. She has yet to be able to take them out because of the resultant arthritis and weakness in her jaw, as she is not able to get her mouth open wide enough for the extractions. My mom also had significant pressure and stress in her childhood, being the eldest sibling in her home. Growing up, she very much felt like the workhorse/maid/nanny rather than an authentically loved individual. That conditioning and perspective still challenges her with feelings of perfectionism and vulnerability, and learning to cope with these perspectives is also part of her healing journey.

My mom and grandma's stories demonstrate our genes' expression is a pool of possibility, rather than a predetermined outcome, depending what conditions the genes are exposed to. While my grandma has now passed on, my mom continues to embark on her journey of wellness through discovering root causes and the related levels of healing, as each of us need to do.

Summary

In homeopathy we call your inherent weaknesses, your "inherited miasms" – the family blueprint that will determine what diseases you will manifest, *if* the conditions are the same as our ancestors with those diseases. I believe genetic diseases seem to be diagnosed frequently in family members not just because we inherit genes, but primarily due to the fact that we also inherit our diets, lifestyles, behaviours, belief systems and even our family traumas. All of these factors affect the three critical areas of our cell development:

1. Nucleus of genes (blueprints)
2. Cell membrane (brain sensor)
3. Mitochondria (energy factories)

Although we can't change our genetic predispositions, we can change the environment those cells are exposed to – toxins, nutrition levels, even the way we feel about things – as these all influence the function and genetic expression of our cells. Statistically, Bruce Lipton actually attributes genetic abnormalities to only be related to 2% of illness. That means our lifestyle controls up to 98%! Now it's time for us to own that percent and rock it!

TWO

Nutrient Deficiencies

"Let food be thy medicine and medicine be thy food."
~ Hippocrates

Mary reported she had been a normal, healthy young woman for most of her life; however, with her impending wedding coming up, the stress was piling up. She first started to feel a slight fluttering of her heart (that admittedly had been a common occurrence for many years). In the past few months, however, she started to notice this come on with more intensity. Soon she started to experience episodes almost daily of heaviness in the body, dizziness, headaches, tingling in her hands, and a racing heart. She would generally feel quite disconnected and "out of it." She had been to the hospital on more than one occasion, and had both stress tests and a Holter monitor. These showed her heart rate would in fact elevate in times of high stress, to around 100 beats per minute. She had a history of hypoglycemia, and had even fainted in the past from not eating consistently. She also reported stomach upset, burping and even pain after eating. She was at a loss of what to eat that would not cause an upset stomach. Her energy was crashing and her anxiety was increasing over the whole ordeal. When we met she was quite concerned, as her health was not improving.

In a world where the vast majority of people in developed countries have more than enough food, it seems like an oxymoron to think we could have nutrient deficiencies. How can we be lacking in our essential nutrients, vitamins, minerals, essential fats and amino acids, with all of the advances in farming practices, accessibility to food year round, and availability of multiple food varieties? Well, there are several reasons why we are still experiencing nutrient deficiencies, despite assumptions being made (even by doctors) that it's a thing of the past. We'll explore these reasons later in the chapter, after a look at the different types of nutrient deficiencies.

I am often surprised at the number of patients that come into my office deficient in one nutrient or another. Most commonly iron and B12 deficiencies are recognized, as these nutrient levels can be easily checked on a blood test by your conventional doctor. However, many nutrients are not well screened via blood work, so often get missed. Think of your blood as a reservoir, or source of nutrients, for your cells. Since the reservoir is deep, by the time you are seeing a nutrient deficiency on blood work, the body's cells have been long starved of that nutrient. It is a big reason why physicians do not conventionally test blood iron as an iron screening test anymore – but rather test ferritin, the storage form of iron. If our storage levels go down, it is an earlier indicator that the iron levels are in jeopardy of becoming significantly deficient very soon.

Interestingly, the numbers for what is considered a B12 deficiency anemia have also changed in value. For years in Canada, when I would run a B12 level in blood, anything over 300 picograms(pg) per millilitre was never reported, as this was considered normal and unnecessary. It got to the point where I wouldn't even run the test and just rely on red blood cell information, because I felt this test was so limited. In 2015, however, labs began reporting the actual B12 values, something that has been done internationally for decades. Japan raised its B12 reference ranges to 500-1300 pg/ml back in the 1980s![2] I believe this range is a more reasonable representation of optimal B12. Yet still in Canada, even though the values are now at least being reported, B12 deficiency is only diagnosed if your value is below 150 pg/ml. It would seem that you basically have to be completely, clinically symptomatic with pernicious anemia before it is considered a treatable value!

There is a suggestion that newer tests like holoTC will be a better B12 test, much like ferritin for iron, in determining actual deficiency.[3] Until this changes and/or B12 references ranges are re-evaluated, the reality is many people will continue to go untreated for B12 deficiencies. Because of its link to energy and nerve function, I believe B12 deficiency should always be evaluated with a combination of blood tests and examination of symptoms, as illustrated in Mary's case:

Based on Mary's symptoms and in-office testing, I quickly inferred that we needed to get her cortisol (a stress hormone) down, and start supporting her nutritionally. I believed a lack of B12 and folic acid was contributing to her numbness, and that the episodes of dizziness and a racing heart were due to being low in potassium, magnesium and trace minerals. Her stress and resultant poor digestion was leading to some significant nutrient deficiencies. We started her on some simple digestive support of apple cider vinegar and bitters before meals to assist in her assimilation of nutrients. We added a multimineral, electrolytes, and B12/folic acid injections weekly, as well as a remedy to address her high cortisol. On her next visit, six weeks later, the numbness was gone, her energy had significantly improved, she was sleeping well, her digestion was much better, and she was feeling notably calmer. She even stopped having the frequent episodes of heart racing. She has since found that as long as she keeps her stress managed and her digestion supported, she doesn't experience these progressively debilitating symptoms that had been plaguing her for years.

Based on my understanding of the effects each nutrient has on our body's function, as well as supportive testing where available, I was able to treat Mary by providing the specific nutrients she needed. Clinical symptoms, however, are just as important – especially when almost every country, and even each state and province, offer different reference ranges for our blood work. Therefore, I will typically only use blood work for B12, Iron and Vitamin D. For other nutrients, we need alternate methods of assessment. I have used private labs for additional testing – from RBC nutrients to hair analysis of minerals – but these tests can be costly, which is often quite prohibitive. Many of the safer nutrients I will dose based on symptoms rather than always relying on testing.

Here are some examples of nutrients with related symptoms, as well as common sources:

Nutrient	Deficiency symptom	Good Sources
B1 (Thiamine)	• Headache • Nausea • Fatigue • Irritability • Abdominal discomfort • Depression • Intolerance to carbohydrates • Beriberi	• Pork • Beef • Poultry • Organ meats • Legumes • Nuts • Nutritional yeast
B2 (Riboflavin)	• Fatigue • Slow growth • Cracks in corner of mouth • Anemia • Eye concerns • Digestive problems • Sore throat • Slowed cellular metabolism	• Dairy • Eggs • Dark green leafy vegetables • Buckwheat • Fish • Poultry • Fortified grains
B3 (Niacin)	• Muscle weakness • Indigestion • Fatigue • Canker sores • Depression • Skin disorders • Pellagra	• Nutritional yeast extract • Rice bran • Liver, pork, beef, chicken, fish • Avocado • Sunflower seeds • Green peas • Mushrooms
B5 (Pantothenic Acid)	• Low Red Blood Cell count • Stress intolerance • Fatigue	• Meats • Egg yolks • Salmon • Lentils, legumes • Nuts and seeds

Nutrient	Deficiency symptom	Good Sources
B6 (Pyridoxine)	• Depression • Tremors • Insomnia • Confusion • Anxiety • Fatigue	• Meats: poultry, fish • Soy • Avocados • Bananas • Carrots • Whole grain flours, brown rice

Nutrient	Deficiency symptom	Good Sources
B9 (Folic Acid)	• Anemia • Restless leg syndrome • Fatigue • Insomnia • Cardiovascular disease • Neural tube defects	• Tomato juice • Beans • Green vegetables

Nutrient	Deficiency symptom	Good Sources
B12 (Cobalamin)	• Anemia • Fatigue • Peripheral neuropathy • Depression • Dementia • Poor memory • Sores at corners of mouth	• Red meats • Nutritional yeast • Algae, greens • Molasses

Nutrient	Deficiency symptom	Good Sources
Vitamin C	• Bleeding gums • Loss of appetite • Fatigue • Slow wound healing • Easy bruising	• Papaya • Orange • Broccoli • Strawberries • Green peppers • Grapefruit

Nutrient	Deficiency symptom	Good Sources
Vitamin D	• Multiple Sclerosis • Poor bone health • Lowered immune function • Hypothyroid	• Produced in skin from UV exposure • Milk • Egg yolk • Liver • Fish

Nutrient	Deficiency symptom	Good Sources
Vitamin A	• Immune function • Eyesight • Growth of skin, hair, nails • Skin rashes, acne	• Beef liver • Sweet potatoes • Carrots • Spinach • Dandelion greens

Nutrient	Deficiency symptom	Good Sources
Vitamin E	• Slow wound healing • Skin disorders • PMS • Heart disease	• Vegetable oils • Wheat germ • Liver • Eggs • Nuts and seeds • Avocados • Asparagus
Vitamin K	• Excessive bleeding • Increased bruising • Heavy periods	• Made in the digestive tract from healthy bacteria • Leafy greens like spinach and kale • Soy • Broccoli
Omega 3	• Dry skin, hair • Peeling brittle nails • Sleep problems • Mood disorders • Poor memory and focus	• Hemp or Flax seeds • Oily fish • Shellfish • Krill oil
Omega 6	• Increased inflammation • Poor memory and focus • Allergies • Dry skin, hair, nails	• Primrose oil • Borage oil • Black currant oil • Vegetables oils (corn, grapeseed, soy, sunflower, cotton seed, safflower, peanut, walnut, sesame)
Calcium	• Muscle cramps • Irritability and anxiety • Osteoporosis	• Dairy • Wheat/soy flour • Molasses • Brazil nuts • Broccoli • Leafy greens • Oysters • Sardines • Salmon
Magnesium	• Nausea and vomiting • Fatigue • Cramps and heart palpitations • Numbness • Seizures	• Green vegetables • Beans • Peas • Nuts and seeds • Whole grains

Nutrient	Deficiency symptom	Good Sources
Chromium	• Blood sugar dysregulation • Insulin resistance • Bone loss • Weakness and fatigue • Poor memory and focus • Poor skin health • Reduced eye health	• Brewer's yeast • Whole grains • Seafood • Broccoli • Prunes • Nuts • Potatoes • Meat

Selenium	• Sore muscles • Decreased thyroid function • RBC loss • Fatigue • Hair loss • Brain fog	• Brewer's yeast • Liver • Butter • Fish and shellfish • Garlic • Sunflower seeds • Brazil nuts

Copper	• Osteoporosis • Anemia • Hair loss • Weakness • Diarrhea • Increased infection • Allergy	• Oysters • Seeds • Leafy greens • Dried legumes • Whole grains and oats • Shellfish • Chocolate • Soy

Iron	• Anemia • Fatigue and weakness • Chest pain • Cold hands and feet • Sore tongue • Brittle nails • Hair loss	• Liver • Red meat • Brewer's yeast • Beans • Spinach • Raisins • Sunflower seeds, nuts

Zinc	• Slow growth and healing • Hair loss • Diarrhea • Low fertility • Eye and skin lesions • Loss of taste • Fatigue	• Red meat • Poultry • Beans • Nuts and pumpkin seeds • Seafood and oysters • Whole grains • Dairy

Why are we seeing more deficiencies?

FOOD PRODUCTION:

The food we eat is a product of our methods of food growth and manufacturing, which are major contributors to a lack of nutrients in our food. Traditional farming used to involve the rotation of crops, and regular use of manure to allow for the soils to maintain their minerals. These methods not only allowed food to maintain essential nutrients such as nitrogen and phosphorus, but also trace minerals, like selenium and manganese. In newer commercial farming, the methods involve actually planting the same crop over and over and using intense fertilizers to get those crops to grow. This leaves the soils stripped of the trace minerals over years and years of growth.

There have been several studies that have been done, including the Davis study in December 2004 in the Journal of the American College of Nutrition, which showed forty-three different vegetables from 1950-1999 with reliable declines in protein, calcium, phosphorus, iron, B2 and Vitamin C. Since the 1940s, increases in crop yields by fertilizers, irrigation and other environmental means have tended to decrease the concentration of minerals in plants.[4]

STATISTICS

- *Since 1940, potatoes have lost 47% of their copper, 45% iron and 35% calcium*
- *Tomatoes have had a 25% drop in calcium, 90% in copper*[5]
- *Another analysis by the Globe and Mail suggested that potatoes dropped 100% of their vitamin A, 57% of vitamin C and 28% of calcium*[6]
- *Broccoli, in a Canadian analysis, showed calcium falling 63% and iron 34%*
- *Canadian data showed that overall, 80% of foods tested on the government food tables over 50 years dropped in calcium and iron. 75% of foods dropped in vitamin A and 50% dropped in vitamin C and B2*[7]

There are multiple analyses that say our food has less nutritional value than it should – however, the responsibility for why this is happening has not been agreed upon. There have also been numerous studies that have shown the nutrient quantities are far superior in organic farming, which by definition uses more traditional practices.

Organic produce is really the best option to ensure we can get as much nutrition out of our food as possible in this day and age. Organic produce can mean higher prices, often not because it costs more to produce, but rather due to the absence of farmer subsidies. However, we vote with our dollars, so as consumers, the more we demand organic, the more available it becomes across grocery stores at affordable prices. Organic produce being found only at the farmer's markets or health food stores has thankfully become a thing of the past. More and more retailers are seeing the value both for our health and their sales. If organic isn't available, don't discount growing your own garden with organically produced seeds and natural gardening practices. This requires a bit of work, but there is nothing like getting to consume the harvests of your labour!

In addition to the concerns around soil stripping, I would venture to say that the next most important production concern is the issue of picking crops before they are fully ripe. Maximization of nutrient content occurs at peak ripening, but because food is often widely distributed, it is picked earlier to prevent ripening before arriving at its destination. This means the longer it took for that grub to go from the ground or tree to our mouths, the more potential for degradation of the vitamins and minerals. Eating from local farms and distributers can curb this loss.

Finally, let's not forget about how we prepare the food. High heat often destroys the nutrients in the food. It can even make it more toxic or rancid for our consumption – think of fried foods or barbequing, for example. The more you can eat fruits, vegetables, dairy and nuts/seeds in a raw state, the more likely you will sustain their nutrients.

Seasonally though, you may want to divert from just eating raw foods, especially in colder climates. The benefit of warm foods in colder climates is well-known in Chinese medicine, as supportive to your Chi or energy flow. We always want to eat cooling foods in the summer and warming foods in the winter, so heating may be a valuable tool in the colder seasons. Some better methods for warming foods can include dehydration, steaming, slow roasting or low heat cooking. One of my favorite cooking methods is using a vacuum method, such as in Saladmaster® pots. Not only are these pots non-leaching of the toxins that are present in most cookware, but they allow for low heat cooking. I love cooking green beans in these pots; in a few short minutes when they are done cooking to perfection, they are still bright green and crunchy, with very minimal water and no oils. I generally don't recommend boiling vegetables especially (unless making bone broths or soups) as you lose much of the nutrients into the water.

NUTRIENT ABSORPTION:

Digestive complaints are probably one of the number one concerns that I see when new patients come into my office: heartburn, indigestion, stomach pain, nausea, bloating, gas and of course constipation or diarrhea. Many people have suffered from these symptoms for years. When I take a medical history, it is all too often that people describe having these symptoms for as long as they can remember! It's so common people often assume them to be normal.

Jill came into my office with some serious digestive complaints. She recalled that as a child, she often had stomach aches and chronic constipation, but it seemed to come and go. However, in the last eight years, after the birth of her two children, she had noticed episodic heartburn that was intensifying. Her MD prescribed an anti-acid, which for a time seemed to help her, but now didn't seem to be making much difference. She was often getting heartburn, belching, indigestion and most recently, periodic diarrhea, something she hadn't ever experienced before. She had tried to change her diet, eliminating a few things, most notably gluten, but it only made a moderate improvement. She felt like there may be more foods she was reacting to, but couldn't pinpoint anything specifically. She was extremely bloated at the end of each day, so much so that she felt like she was four months pregnant. She was also finding her energy to be really low, and could hardly get out of bed in the morning. She reported restless legs at night and fairly regular tension headaches. She felt wiped out and at a loss for what to do.

What was going on with Jill? The end result of inflammation in the gut is an increased intestinal permeability or leaky gut – but before we go there, let's start at the top to understand how this all happens.

Digestion, as with all the intricately designed systems in the body, has been perfectly created for the function it provides – extracting nutrition from our food and eliminating waste. This function requires that we support it in the right ways: chew our food properly, don't drink a lot of fluids with our meals, don't multitask when we eat, and of course be in a relaxed state when we're eating. The reason for this is that we need to be in a calm state, otherwise known as a parasympathetic state, for proper digestive function. The parasympathetic nervous system is required to support blood flow, nerve stimulation, and enzyme secretion for the purpose of breaking down your food and extracting those building blocks the body needs for survival.

Since many people cannot consistently support proper biological digestion, (never mind worrying about *what* they're actually eating), they can end up having problems. I can't tell you how many patients come into my office on an antacid of some type, prescribed or self-medicated – and in order to return to a healthy gut, it's the first thing I work to take them off. Long term use of antacids will never serve anyone. Only in rare cases where people are taking certain medications like NSAIDS (non-steroidal anti-inflammatory drugs like ibuprophen for example), or for the short term use in treating ulcerations or erosions, will I ever use them in my practice. Your stomach was designed to sustain acid! Believe it or not, it can endure really intense acid, very low on the pH scale.

So what is really happening when our acid production seems to be off? Heartburn is actually a result most commonly of low stomach acid, not high! With normal function, the stomach, when triggered to digest, sets off several automatic functions to get the job done:

1. Initially, when we are smelling and chewing our food, the
   stomach is preparing to digest by getting the juices flowing.

We also release amylase in the saliva that starts the breakdown of our carbohydrates in the mouth.

2. This secretion of stomach acid then stimulates the contraction of the stomach muscle to move the contents around in the stomach, and break those food pieces into smaller particles. This promotes good muscle tone in the stomach so that you are not prone to a hiatal hernia for example.

3. The acids stimulate the release of mucin to protect the lining of the stomach. You actually have your own natural Pepto-Bismol®!

4. The acid also, very importantly, causes the contraction of the cardiac sphincter (valve between the esophagus and stomach) so nothing can come back up (which happens in heartburn)!

5. Acid is also really important for the release of the protein called intrinsic factor, which helps us absorb vitamin B12.

6. The strong acid is also there to kill off pathogens, like viruses or bacteria. Food is not sterile, so this prevents infection from reaching past the stomach.

7. Stomach acid also will eventually stimulate the activation of enzymes in the stomach and duodenum. The pancreatic enzymes lie dormant otherwise, as we don't want those enzymes active all the time and continuing to digest, lest they begin to digest our own tissues!

8. Lastly, the acid also stimulates the release of bicarbonate, to neutralize the acid once it enters the small intestine. The small intestine's role in digestion is for the absorption of our nutrients, vitamins, minerals, amino acids, fats, and carbohydrates. All the building blocks for growth, repair and function are absorbed solely in this section of the digestive tract.

Biologically, there is only one reason why we will naturally reduce our digestive function, and that is age. Over time the amount of hydrochloric acid secreting cells, called parietal cells, decrease. This may be a big reason why the geriatric population is one of the largest population groups to experience nutrient deficiencies. They are the one group where constant stomach acid support and enzyme supplements may be warranted in the long term. The second reason our digestive function can be inhibited is from stress, and not allowing the body to enter into the parasympathetic (relaxed state) when eating. This is common when we eat on the go, standing at the counter, watching TV or in our cars – where we really aren't focused on eating or digesting.

So what happens when proper acid function fails, as it did with Jill? The food just sits in the stomach, causing a person to feel fuller more quickly, and often nauseated. Belching may increase, since the food sits there and ferments in the stomach. There may even be food contents that come back up in the throat, as the cardiac sphincter does not contract – regurge, anyone? If that goes on long enough, then we might see esophageal erosions (pain) and scar tissue (difficulty swallowing). Since pathogens (aka problematic microbes) may not be killed off effectively either, they may make their way down to the intestines, possibly colonizing and creating infection – aka more inflammation and damage. It is at this point in the process where Jill was experiencing bloating, gas, chronic constipation, and finally diarrhea. Classically this is often diagnosed as IBS (Irritable Bowel Syndrome).

Also, when the enzymes are not activated, large pieces of food end up in the intestine and are not fully broken down into the amino acids, glucose, fatty acids, vitamins, and minerals our bodies need. At this point, people often supplement with enzymes which allow them to digest better, but generally speaking, I actually disagree with this. I reserve enzymes for severely compromised digestive systems. Otherwise, with continued use, they may suppress your own enzyme production – and by what I have just described, the main aspect of the problem is not that you don't have enzymes, rather that you're not activating them.

With Jill, we can now see how the lack of stomach acid, likely from years of poor digestive habits and the ongoing stress of juggling work and family life, caused her suppressed digestive function and the resulting heartburn and other digestive problems. When her cardiac sphincter was too relaxed, the juices from the stomach (which are always going to be more acidic than the esophagus) rose and caused the burning sensation. And although the antacids initially gave her relief by simply neutralizing all her acid (but not preventing it from coming up), they in fact made the whole digestive picture worse on the long term.

Now with all these stressors in her life, what was Jill left with after eating? A largely undigested meal was entering the small intestine, with no effective way to break it down further, and the possibility of a whole host of unfriendly microorganisms coming along for the ride. The result: inflammation. A full on battlefield in the lower abdomen – compromised gut flora (killing off the good bacteria), digestion of the food by abnormal microorganisms (bloating and gas), and irritation to the gut lining from the toxins produced in this process (leaky gut).

The accumulated effect of all this irritation is increased intestinal permeability and damage. Imagine your small intestine is like a cheese cloth – it allows some tiny elements through (glucose, amino acids, vitamins, etc.) – but provides a barrier for most other elements (whole proteins, toxins or carbohydrate chains). Then imagine having tears in that cheese cloth. That is leaky gut. More substances, including whole food particles, can leak through the intestinal barrier.

This repetitive whole food particle absorption is what leads to food reactions. Your body will look at a dairy protein, or soy protein, or whatever you're exposing your body to the most, and say, "Foreign invader! We don't know what this is, get rid of it! Attack!" Then, the delayed hypersensitivity reaction is born, or as some call it, food sensitivities. We get an onslaught of antibodies, immunoglobulin G (IgG) specifically, to remember to clear that invader as soon as it comes into contact, and now we have a food intolerance.

Due to the developed sensitivity to gluten, Jill noticed improvement with gluten elimination, but not a total resolution of her stomach issues. The food intolerance was a **result** *of the digestive process breakdown, not the other way around. This is why it is so important that we never just stop at eliminating the problem foods. The gut must be healed as well. In Jill's case, because the gut was damaged, symptoms like diarrhea and bloating started to show up even after the gluten elimination. After years of dysfunctional digestion, she had developed infection in her intestines – which also contributed to irregular bowels, and further possible food allergies. Her other symptoms, from fatigue to restless leg and even headaches, resulted from the compromised absorption of nutrients and excess inflammation in the body.*

To resolve Jill's stomach issues, we had to start at the beginning. First, we tested for and removed all reactive foods, and treated an infection of abnormal bacteria (SIBO – small intestine bacterial overgrowth). Second, we worked to heal the gut and esophagus by working with digestive healing supplements (with L-glutamine, deglycerated licorice, Marshmallow root, and Slippery Elm). And third, we retrained her stomach to secrete acid with a betaine HCl challenge and promoted normal healthy flora in the gut with probiotics. This process of digestive restoration can take months, and sometimes the food eliminations have to be indefinite, depending on the severity of the situation. But ultimately, as the gut is where so much of our immune function lies, it is imperative to stop the cycle of inflammation and the development of further food allergies.

Jill's case is not unique. The above case and healing process literally describes almost every digestive problem that I see in my office – variations being simply that different symptoms dominate in different people. The symptoms can include cramping, bloating, belching, diarrhea and constipation. This digestive dysfunction can be associated to diseases from IBS (Irritable Bowel Syndrome), Crohn's, Colitis, GERD (Gastroesophageal Reflux Disease), diverticulitis, appendicitis and digestive infections, as well as several other diseases that don't manifest in the gut but are a result of its breakdown – like acne, eczema, sinusitis, environmental allergies, chronic infections, autoimmune diseases and even cancer. 70% to 80% of your immune system's functioning occurs in the gut, from the mouth to the anus, so realistically, every single disease treatment has to include digestive healing. It may not completely resolve the symptoms, since you may have many other root causes you have to address as well, but it is such an important part of the healing process.

So as this abnormal digestive function progresses from stomach to intestine to colon, the constant inflammation significantly affects the absorption of our nutrients. Many people try to reconcile the problem through extensive use of supplements. I hate to say it, but a lot of us just have really expensive poop when we take them. I'm always amazed at the number of women that come into my office, iron deficient for example, despite taking iron supplements for years. The only possible cause, since the *source* is there (providing the supplement is of sufficient quality), is that absorption is compromised.

A Further Note on Food Sensitivities:

Food sensitivities or IgG allergies that result from this leaky gut lining process really stems from all of the root causes of disease. From the dysfunction of our eating habits, to the stress that blocks stomach acid, infections that ensue from improper digestion and repetitive antibiotic use, chemical toxicity associated with food additives and sprays, and irritation from adulterated or genetically modified foods – all of these factors can cause a huge assault on the intestinal lining. This sets the tone for a damaged and dysfunctional gut lining.

Added to that onslaught is the fact that most of us have a limited variety in our diet. Most people eat about ten foods consistently. This leads to repetitive exposure of these food antigens to the immune system, thereby increasing the likelihood that they become allergies. The more often our immune system is exposed to a food antigen that found its way through the gut lining, the more likely we will develop a reaction to it. Hence, the most common foods we eat often end up becoming our worst allergies. The symptoms of food allergies or sensitivities caused by leaky gut can range from digestive pain, to bloating, bowel changes, migraines, weight gain or weight loss, fatigue, muscle pain, or sinus congestion. Environmental allergies may also develop.

In children, I often see food sensitivities manifest as either skin issues like eczema, digestive issues like stomach aches, repetitive infections like the ear or throat, or behavioural/emotional issues like tantrums or insomnia. Behavior is often overlooked because it's not a "digestive" symptom. However, many of our neurotransmitters of the brain are actually formed in the digestive tract, hence the gut can directly affect brain function!

Inherent to these sensitivity problems is not just the food we eat, but what we've done to it. We have largely changed food's molecular makeup like that of genetically modified foods. Wheat has certainly gotten a bad rap as of late, largely due to how it has been adulterated for optimal commercial production. Is it a coincidence that wheat is one of the most common food sensitivities?

Another point to consider is that as when we experience problems with certain foods, we may begin to create psychological attachments around foods as being good or bad. In fact, foods are just supportive or detrimental, but not good or bad. Wheat, in our example above, is not a "bad" food, just a commonly problematic one for those with leaky gut. Yet the fear that can come with eating grains like wheat, may actually have just as much of an impact on their digestion than the wheat itself. Sometimes how we feel about a food can have an effect on us just as much as the modifications to it. This is a concept largely explored by Bruce Lipton, in the study of epigenetics, that we covered in the last chapter.

Many of the foods which a person becomes sensitive to through the leaky gut process may be able to reintroduce into the body after healing is complete – others however, may never be compatible, as food continues to be manipulated in both production and processing. For example, dairy is a very common food sensitivity – however, historically dairy would have been a very rare allergy concern. What has changed? In order to compensate for the mass demand for milk products, and to ensure safety in large production facilities, North America requires homogenization (spin) and pasteurization (flash heat) of milk. These processes were introduced to reduce the incidence of infections from microorganisms in the milk, like salmonella, listeria and E. coli. This law was only enacted roughly fifty years ago, and more strictly enforced for the past twenty-five years in Canada. The result is that all dairy we consume is pasteurized, despite being widely consumed and accepted in raw form worldwide. The possible connection then to a dairy allergy, may in fact be due to the treatment of the milk, rather than milk itself. There are studies that have suggested that children who drank raw milk had significantly lower allergies, asthma and eczema.[8] The treatment process of milk, using pasteurization and homogenization, causes the milk to lack natural healthy microorganisms (probiotics), and denatures the natural enzymes to help us digest it. Again, milk itself may not be the problem – rather, what have we done to it? Perhaps we've traded one problem for another? Certainly something to consider.

NUTRIENT DEPENDENCIES:

While people are generally familiar with the concept of supply and demand when it comes to the commercial market, the concept is more elusive when we talk about our bodies. However, if you think about it, it makes sense that when your body has a higher demand on it – if you're sick, stressed or doing more than your body is used to – your nutritional requirements are higher as well. But we often seem to miss identifying this concept. Here is a common scenario I see in my office – when a person is sick with a cold, I will commonly recommend taking more vitamin C, even to the point of bowel intolerance. It is known that vitamin C absorption is roughly 40% from the gut, and dose dependent. Meaning the more we take, the less we absorb. On any given day, the average person will tolerate approximately 3000-5000 mg per day before the common side effect of diarrhea kicks in. When people are sick, however, it's interesting that they can often tolerate up to 10,000-15,000 mg (dosed as 1000 mg every hour) before diarrhea results. Why could that be? Is it the mere fact that the body's immune system heavily relies on vitamin C, hence when fighting an infection, could require more?

The body is constantly trying to be in balance. It would therefore naturally make sense that when it's working harder – performing those enzymatic reactions more often and burning more energy (remember ATP) – it would need more fuel. All the nutrients that we consume – the vitamins, minerals, fats, and amino acids – are the building blocks and fuel of life for our physical selves. They are the keys to unlocking all of the actions we need to make our body work, and when the demand is up, the supply must also follow. Sometimes this can come from storage forms of these nutrients in the body – like vitamin A or D from the liver, amino acids from our muscles, or calcium from our bones – but if this process goes on consistently and chronically, and we are not filling up our reserves, the tanks get low.

Stress is a common example of how our body systems use the concept of supply and demand. When we undergo periods of stress, we ramp up the use of our energy molecules, as well as increase our cortisol production. Cortisol is a hormone secreted from the adrenal glands in these times of stress. This naturally leads to the requirement of more nutrients to foster that increased demand – nutrients like magnesium, vitamin C and B vitamins. Hence, the B vitamins are often one of the nutrients to become low in the body with chronic stress, and, because they are used in so many different areas in the body, a deficiency can lead to diffuse and vague symptoms. Those symptoms can include fatigue, mental fogginess, changes in brain chemistry and moods, or changes in menstrual cycles and hormones, just to name a few. All are common systems that I am sure most of us have experienced when stress has been higher at different times in our lives.

Another interesting example of our nutritional conundrum: North America has one of the highest osteoporosis levels in the world, yet we are amongst the top dairy consumers in the world. How can that be? Well, understand that as we enter into our thirties, we stop building bone and then our bodies just work to maintain bone density.[9] So any conditions that cause leaching of calcium out of our bones will lead to loss in bone density, despite appropriate levels of consumption. Dairy is high in calcium, which is good, but the challenge is that dairy is also very acid forming in the body. Dairy, along with grains, meats, alcohol and caffeine, are our main acid formers – and are also staples in the classic North American diet. This excess of acidity increases the necessity for our body to buffer the change in pH in our blood and tissues using the reserve minerals our body has already stored – like magnesium, phosphorus and calcium. Therefore, the calcium from dairy has little impact on the total calcium reserves in the body as it is just used as a buffer. Maintaining an alkaline diet to preserve an optimum neutral pH level in the system would go much further towards maintaining bone health than just taking a calcium supplement. That would reduce the demand for calcium to act as a buffer to the excess acid, and therefore keep it in the bones. Good alkaline foods include lemons, limes, avocados, yams, onions, kale, broccoli, green tea, beets, grapes and lettuce, to name a few. Most fruits and vegetables fall into the alkaline category.

Unless we can compensate for the increased demand for nutrients due to imbalances in the body, symptoms will always ensue. Symptoms are your body's way of saying, "Hey! Pay attention here." They send a message with the goal of getting the body back into balance – to give it the very things it needs to work. Nutrients are not optional – they are a fundamental necessity of life. Choosing the right foods and supplements is really a question of what our body demands right now, not just our choice flavours. We will examine ways of treating nutritional deficiencies, in a holistic manner, in Chapter 7 – First Level of Healing: The Physical Body.

Just as an athlete eats sufficient calories before a race to anticipate the increased energy demand, so should we all anticipate the demands of our bodies when we are under different circumstances, ages, and conditions than usual. Every wonder why we have cravings? That is another symptom to pay attention to – trying to understand why we always want more sugar, not just ignoring or giving into it. Is it that my body is needing more energy? My blood sugar is imbalanced? My stress is high? Is it that I have an infection, like yeast, taking up my sugar supply? These are the little signals that we are constantly getting from our system to try to keep us in balance. You have the ability to tap into your body and any symptoms showing up at any moment. Just take a moment and turn your focus inside. What shows up? These tools you are learning will give you more awareness of what is going on inside. You have the power to know and heal your body when you truly pay attention to it.

Summary

Just as your car requires oil to function properly, nutrients are required for all physical functions of the body. Imagine if you didn't consume enough nutrients – it's like not putting oil in your car...You might drive for a little while, possibly creating some damage to that car, but eventually it simply won't run. The body is our vehicle, and it's imperative we give it all the essential tools it needs to work properly. This fundamental root cause is significantly important, as recent changes in society dictate that:

1. Our food supply is ever changing. We lose many nutrients due to food production, distribution and preparation.
2. Our bodies are experiencing more exposures to toxins and stress which can create further digestive damage and dysfunction. Nutrient absorption is therefore compromised.
3. Our lifestyles are more demanding. We may not be meeting the needs of our body, hence also leading to nutrient deficiencies.

Being informed and advocating a simple and clean way of eating is essential. It's getting back to basics, so that our God given ability to utilize for sustenance the very things that are all around us – whole and healthy foods – is optimized. Shift your paradigm to thinking of healthy food as being a necessity to thrive, not just to survive. Which would you rather do?

THREE

Toxicity

"Human use of fossil fuels is altering the chemistry of the atmosphere; oceans are polluted and depleted of fish; 80 percent of Earth's forests are heavily impacted or gone yet their destruction continues. An estimated 50,000 species are driven to extinction each year. We dump millions of tonnes of chemicals, most untested for their biological effects, and many highly toxic, into air, water and soil. We have created an ecological holocaust. Our very health and survival are at stake, yet we act as if we have plenty of time to respond."
~ *David Suzuki*

"We are living on the planet as if we have another one to go to."
~ *Terry Swearingen*

In understanding toxins, we must first understand the extent of the problem. Toxicity is a global problem that we are all facing. Leaders like David Suzuki have been talking to the public about the environment for decades, but very few of us have actually realized what the destruction and toxicity of our environment means to our health. In this chapter, I want you to fully understand the impact and what is really at stake.

When people hear the word toxicity, they often imagine hazmat suits and a major toxic chemical spill with people being quarantined. And while there have been multiple examples of oil spills from train derailments almost annually, very few of us actually think about the daily, insidious exposure that we are bathed in each and every day from the toxic soup of chemicals used on our body, on our food and in our environment. Because we often cannot smell or see toxins, most people rarely think they have any exposures. Recognizing what a toxin is therefore, is the first step in this awareness.

Although for simplicity I will only use the term toxin throughout this book, I want you to understand the difference between the commonly used term toxin, and the more official term toxicant. A toxicant by definition is just a toxic or poisonous substance. In popular usage, the term is often used to denote substances made by humans or introduced into the environment by human activity, in contrast to *toxins*, which are only "toxicants produced naturally by a living organism."[10] So what we can deduce from this definition is that a toxicant is actually something that is natural *or* man-made that can cause harm to the body. Hence, although a toxicant is the broader term, toxin is the more commonly used and understood term.

Some examples of natural toxins are things like snake venom, bacterial toxins or free radicals. Man-made ones may include pesticides, herbicides, flavourings, preservatives, artificial colours, plastics and so on. There are well over 80,000 man-made chemicals in use in the US alone, with the US Department of Health estimating more than 2000 new ones introduced each year, most of which are not actually tested for their long-term health effects.[11] These are in addition to the naturally occurring toxins as mentioned in the examples above. Alarming!

What does this mean to our bodies? Thankfully, we have been divinely engineered to handle toxins, primarily thanks to our liver, kidneys, colon, lymphatic systems, and skin:

1. The liver filters the toxins, changing them from a fat soluble

form to a water soluble one we can eliminate.
2. The kidneys remove the toxins from the blood into urine.
3. The colon removes toxins from the digestive tract and the liver through bile in the form of stool.
4. The lymphatics clear the cellular garbage and move it to the corresponding processing areas like the spleen.
5. The skin releases fat soluble toxins through your pores via perspiration.

However, the success of this detoxification system was based on what mother nature could throw at us, not man-made additions! It becomes a problem for your health when you have an *excess intake of toxins from the environment,* or *excess production of toxins in the body from microbes or cellular metabolism,* and/or a *reduced elimination out of the body.* If any of these situations occur, the resultant overload of toxins becomes stored in the body. They're typically sequestered in fat and bone tissue, where they can remain for many years and be damaging to cells – even at low doses.

We simply were not designed to deal with the level of toxins our bodies are being exposed to today. They are literally found in every-thing in our world of convenience. There are estimates that we are exposed to hundreds of thousands of man-made chemicals each and every single day.

Think of how your day goes: from waking up in the morning, eating, travelling, working, and so on. Your daily routine. Here is a simplified example of some common exposures:

1. The sheets, towels and clothing you use each day (laundry soaps, fabric softeners, dryer sheets)
2. The mattress and bedding you are sleeping on (laundry soaps, fabric softeners, fire retardants, PVCs)
3. Taking a shower (soaps, shampoos, conditioners, chlorine in the tap water)
4. Getting ready for the day (lotions, hair products, deodorants, perfumes, toothpaste, cosmetics – on average, US women are exposed to 168 chemicals daily through their use of 12 different personal products/cosmetics [12]
5. Eating breakfast, lunch and dinner (processed? genetically modified? sprayed with chemicals? what is it packaged in? how was it cooked or prepared?)
6. Driving to/from work (plastic off-gassing in the car, exhaust)
7. Work day (office building? dealing with receipts? plastics? cleaners or chemicals?)
8. Going home and going to bed (similar exposures as above)

Above is an example of just one day, but what if we also add in the fact that we may live in a community with air pollution, from a mine, mill or factory, or close to golf courses or farms/orchards? What if we frequently fly, and are being exposed to high levels of jet fuel and radiation? Or what about if we are living in a newer home with off-gassing from paints, cupboards, glues, or flooring – or maybe an old home with lead paints or pipes, asbestos or molds? Or perhaps we also drink alcohol, smoke or have smoked cigarettes, or have had mercury amalgam fillings. Other potential sources of toxins: we have been vaccinated, we eat fish or seafood, we chew gum, we have gas appliances, we eat fast foods, we clean our house...these all have the potential for toxicity! As you can see, the unfortunate reality is that there is no escaping toxins. This is what I call the 21st century condition. Our only option is to become aware of what and where they are, and reduce or eliminate all the areas under our control. This is why detoxing and cleansing are not fads, nor weight loss techniques, but they are a mere essential part of living in the 21st century. We will discuss more about the concept of detoxing in Chapter 7 while exploring physical healing.

Although the sheer number of toxins to deal with may feel overwhelming, rest assured there is good news here too. As you become aware of these exposures and their impact on your life, you can begin to avoid many of them, make new choices and advocate for a cleaner, safer world. Visualize what a cleaner world would look like to you. You have more power than you think to create it. Not only can you "reduce, reuse and recycle," but you can make the biggest impact by choosing where you spend your money. Choose companies that fight to maintain the same ideals you value: environmental sustainability, waste reduction, and materials that are non-toxic, organic and non-genetically modified.

How do I know if toxins are an issue for me?

As you probably can guess, I am going to say toxins are an issue for everyone, but let's talk more about the specifics. It is more common than I would like to see in my office, but often patients come in with a myriad of toxicity symptoms. So much so, we have even classified one related diagnosis as *"Multiple Chemical Sensitivities,"* which really just means toxic overload.

General Symptoms	Associated illnesses	Toxic effects
▪ Fatigue ▪ Constipation or Diarrhea ▪ Headaches ▪ Skin rashes ▪ Joint pain ▪ Chronic pain ▪ Sinus congestion ▪ Water retention ▪ Disturbed sleep	▪ Fibromyalgia ▪ Chronic Pain ▪ Obesity ▪ Auto-immune disease ▪ Chronic infections (e.g. Lyme) ▪ Skin conditions ▪ Allergies ▪ Liver disease ▪ Chronic Fatigue ▪ Fertility issues ▪ Cancer	▪ Irritation ▪ Inflammation ▪ Enzyme blocking ▪ Free radical production ▪ Blocked nutrient absorption ▪ Slow healing ▪ Persistent bruising ▪ Tissue breakdown ▪ Aging ▪ Hormone inactivity (e.g. thyroid)

How do toxins get into our bodies?

There are three main routes for toxins to enter our bodies – through what we put in our mouth, what we put on our skin, and what we breathe in the air. These three types are our environmental toxins or exotoxins.

There is a fourth source of toxins as well – endotoxins, which naturally are created by the bacterial microbiome in our bodies. A certain amount of endotoxins are normally produced with our symbiotic or helpful microorganisms; however, if that microflora becomes imbalanced, through infections or antibiotics, those toxic levels may increase and cause problems. However, I will focus on exotoxins in this chapter as we will be focusing on ways to control our exposure to them.

Ideally, toxins will only ever enter our bodies through our digestive tracts, lungs and skin, because those tissues were created with some filtering capacity. Hence, they will certainly try to prevent the absorption of toxins. However, if any of these areas are compromised with inflammation or damage, their ability to selectively filter some toxins may also be compromised. A common example would be leaky gut syndrome as discussed in the previous chapter – since the intestinal lining is damaged, it becomes more permeable and likely to absorb more toxins.

If toxins make it through our defenses and enter the body, they absorb into the extracellular matrix. This includes the blood, the connective tissues and the lymphatic system. One of the most important areas to focus on in cleansing is the lymphatics, as this network remove toxins from the cells. If excessive toxins are housed in the body, disease and dysfunction begin. The toxins can then damage the cellular components and affect their function; thereby causing, for all intents and purposes, a sick cell.

Once in the system, toxins will be streamlined by the body to the organs that can filter it. Largely, they continue to the liver, where they are broken down through two phases of detoxification. The purpose of this, is so that the liver can create a less damaging water soluble version of the toxin from a fat soluble form. This allows for ease of elimination – most commonly through the kidneys or the colon. The skin and lungs can also help in the removal role as well! But when overloaded, not all toxins are able to be removed this way.

How can I control what toxins I'm exposed to?

1) FOOD

When little three-year-old Sammy came to see me, he could hardly stand to be in his own skin. He had severe eczema all over his body – his ears, face, hands, arm creases, groin and legs. He was incessantly itchy. His parents reported that he always seemed irritable, and wasn't sleeping well. They were also noticing some behavioral problems both at daycare, where he was pinching other kids, and at home, where he was having tantrums. His parents were frustrated and confused. The cortisone creams they were using only seemed to give him temporary relief, and often worsened the rash in the long run. They were desperate.

Upon listening to his history, his parents reported he was a vaginally delivered baby, so I knew he had a good first exposure to mom's healthy vaginal bacteria when he was born, helping to colonize his gut. This is not the case in C-section babies, though fortunately more doctors and midwives are adopting the practice of swabbing the mother's vaginal canal to introduce the needed bacteria to these babies' mouths once they are born- simple and ingenious!

Sammy's mom, however, had a tough time nursing and felt she wasn't able to produce enough milk, so he was switched over to formula at about three weeks of age. This meant he didn't get the continued exposure to his mom's healthy flora and helpful antibodies that were present in her breast milk. She had noticed he was a bit colicky as an infant, and seemed to suffer from constipation around five months of age, when they started to introduce solid foods. They did the food introductions as her doctor recommended, with a grain cereal first and then some vegetables, but quickly moved on to introduce most varieties of foods by about ten months of age. He would get the odd rash then, but it seemed to have gotten much worse over the years.

Because of Sammy's early nutritional sources, my first thoughts were that his rash was a result of potential toxicity and ultimately reactions to certain foods. At that very young age, his highly permeable intestine would be more susceptible to poor food quality and toxicity than an adult with a strong, fully developed gut. Unfortunately, not all food is created equal, and the way we produce food today has changed a great deal over the last century, and even more so in the last forty years.

With the onset of commercial farming, we have drastically changed the production, composition, and consumption patterns of our food. Where it was once commonplace to live on or be close to a family run farm, we have now primarily switched to large farm factories of produce and animals. While we have improved efficiencies in food production with newer equipment, many of the newer practices have left our food supply worse off.

Commercial farming started on a large scale after World War II, when chemical warfare companies no longer had a war to focus on, so concentrated their efforts on chemical warfare on our plants to control weeds that competed with crops. This meant heavy spraying of chemicals over the decades including DDT, PCBs and Agent Orange. Many of these, thankfully, have since been banned from many countries around the world due to human harm. The initial problem was that these chemicals were so toxic, they killed everything! So, in order to continue the use of these products (like glyphosate, i.e. Roundup®), the next step was to make foods immune to these toxins through genetic adulteration. An ingenious plan, a seed that is entirely dependent on the use of a pesticide! Now these crops didn't die from the excessive spraying of glyphosate, but were completely covered in this highly toxic chemical and ready for consumption. In turn, we got to eat the toxin!

But it didn't stop there; chemical companies continued to unnaturally and invasively introduce selected gene characteristics to create "superfoods." However, unlike the historical practices of species cross-pollination or grafting, they decided to inject the genetic makeup from completely different organisms into first plants, and then even animals. Since when did God intend for insect or bacterial DNA to be inside our food? What's worse, this unnatural engineering produced strains of species that are virtually impossible for nature to create, leading to a whole host of unpredictable effects in their genetic makeup. The introduction of these unnatural species into our food supply leads to human consumption of unrecognizable proteins with the potential for risks of toxic reactions in the body.

Citing several animal studies, The American Academy of Environmental Medicine concludes "there is more than a casual association between GM foods and adverse health effects" and that "GM foods pose a serious health risk in the areas of toxicology, allergy and immune function, reproductive health, and metabolic, physiologic and genetic health." For example, if the Bt toxin, a genetically engineered bacterial toxin produced in corn, is lethal enough to break apart the digestive tracts of insects, what is it doing to our own digestive tracts when we eat GM corn, or animals that eat GM corn?[13] It is suggested that not enough appropriate studies have been done around GMOs and human health.[14] Therefore, perhaps it is also possible that the incidence of allergies and liver/digestive issues that have been on the rise in the past few decades are also correlated to the introduction of GMOs? [15] [16]

Another problem that results in the increased toxicity of our food supply is the loss of biodiversity. 88% of corn produced in the US (over 80% in Canada) is GM. We can potentially consume up to fifty natural varieties of corn, but we invest heavily in one species instead, making it particularly vulnerable to environmental changes (such as droughts) and organisms (such as new pests, or reduced resistance to existing pests). Do we want all our eggs in one basket? Never in history have we relied so heavily upon one type of species for a primary food source.

With the dominance of commercial farming, we have commonly come to believe that the only way to sustain our increasing population is by relying on practices that involve both the heavy spraying of our foods and the stripping of nutrients from our soil. We rarely consider that the real problem with shortfalls in food supply are not from increasing population demands, but in fact, are from the excesses of the wealthy. In 2005, it was reported that 20% of the world's wealthiest populations consumed 76.6% of the world energy sources, as opposed to the 20% of the poorest population, who consumed 1.5% of the world's energy sources. [17]

Although changing the dietary practices of the rich would certainly be helpful, the majority of food shortfalls in lower income countries occur more from harmful economic systems, effects of conflict, and climate change, rather than simply not employing commercial farming practices.

One common belief is that genetically modifying food increases productivity. However, we also need to consider that the increase in productivity can be potentially attributed to better farming practices and modern technology – as compared to the simpler practices of the 1800s. In fact, if all we did was improve efficiency and reduce waste around what we already produce, we would have more than enough

DR. ALANA BERG, ND

to feed the world. Beginning with the farmer and ending with our forks, we currently lose about 40% of our food to landfills.

It is also baffling how we can assume the government agencies that allow GMOs on the market are there for our sole benefit. Historically, these very organizations that approve GMO use only require the "unbiased" studies right from the companies that want to produce these foods. The problem is, no one can access these seeds for independent study because the patents are owned by the biotech companies. In 2012, a small, long-term, independent study was done in France, where rats fed Roundup®-tolerant genetically modified maize developed massive tumours.[18] After much controversy, however, the publisher forced the study to be retracted. It's a perfect scenario for biotech companies – little resistance to getting questionable food on the market for mass consumption, without the need for labelling or other forms of accountability. If a problem does develop, there is no way to trace it back to the source – and we are all unknowingly consuming these GMOs every day. If they are so safe, why the secrecy? As Henry Kissinger, former US Secretary of State said, "Who controls the food supply controls the people."

To a large degree, GMOs are a mass experiment with a lack of long term studies. I know for myself, I don't want my family to be a part of this mass experiment, and I'd like the basic right to opt out. But until lawmakers and governments are pressured enough to change the current regulations our best option is to look for labels that say non-GMO – or better yet, seek out Certified Organic foods. In order to be deemed organic, the food must also be GMO free. The label of Organic also implies no chemical use, and traditional farming practices (like crop rotation), which allow for increased nutrient content, as well as less toxic burden. Apples to apples, there is no question that the amount of toxins found in organic meat, dairy and produce are much lower, but the foods cannot be 100% toxin-free – the unfortunate reality of our world today is that nothing can be perfectly free of toxins. We can't control how the water flows or how the wind blows, as these lead to contamination of even the best farming practices.

Consciously reducing our toxic food burden, by choosing organic and non-GMO as much as possible, will always be beneficial to our health.

The most common GM foods are:

1. corn (like high fructose corn syrup)
2. soy
3. canola
4. cotton seed
5. beet sugar
6. alfalfa

Added to this list is the new GM "arctic" apple to be grown in the Okanagan, BC, as well as GM salmon and several others working their way onto the market.

The most highly sprayed foods, aka "The Dirty Dozen," that are recommended to be purchased as organic are, in order:

1. apples
2. celery
3. sweet bell peppers
4. peaches
5. strawberries
6. imported nectarines
7. grapes
8. spinach
9. lettuce
10. cucumbers
11. domestic blueberries
12. potatoes (green beans and kale)

Conversely, "The Clean Fifteen" for the least sprayed produce include:

1. avocados
2. sweet corn

3. pineapples
4. cabbage
5. sweet peas (frozen)
6. onions
7. asparagus
8. mangoes
9. papayas (if not GMO)
10. kiwi
11. eggplant
12. honeydew melon
13. grapefruit
14. cantaloupe
15. cauliflower

While these fifteen foods would contain less toxins than "The Dirty Dozen," it would still be beneficial to purchase organic versions of these items, for the reasons outlined above.

Genetically modified, non-organic food played a significant part in Sammy's case. Because we knew his early nutritional background, we decided to do some food testing, in which a dairy casein allergy was discovered. I also recommended the removal of all processed and GMO foods. And finally, I recommended some digestive support through introducing probiotics. Within six weeks, 90% of his skin reactions had completely cleared. He also seemed happier, and everyone in the house was getting much better sleep! His parents were amazed. I recommended they continue to follow a non-GMO diet. We then started to work on digestive healing using homeopathic medicines. After about four months and a food retest, we allowed for some raw dairy cheese to be introduced. Sammy experienced no problems with this, although his mom was very leery about adding anything more. They were so happy their little boy was feeling so good.

This story happens all too commonly in my practice, as the people whose digestive tracks are the most susceptible to toxins in our foods will always be children. Their guts are still forming at a young age and are highly permeable, especially as infants. Therefore, when they get exposed to a variety of types of foods early on - through formula and early food introductions - along with their associated toxins, this can dramatically impact their health and function later on. We all need to be aware of the impact of toxins within our food supply, as they can affect people of all ages.

2) ENVIRONMENTAL

When Kim came to see me, she was not doing well. She initially came in for what she believed were allergies and asthma; however, I realized it was much more than allergies when she began to describe her symptoms. She reported sneezing, coughing, sore throat, poor immune function, repetitive pneumonia, fatigue, swelling, hypoglycemia, diarrhea and heartburn. She even reported vomiting on occasion, which tasted and smelled like bleach. I diagnosed her with Multiple Chemical Sensitivities. She came from Southeast Asia origi-nally, and since English wasn't her first language, was having trouble finding a job that didn't expose her to chemicals. She was currently working in a dry cleaning shop pressing shirts. She was also reacting to carpets and cigarette smoke in her current living condition. Her blood test reported elevated liver enzymes, so I knew her liver was being taxed.

Once we started some gentle detoxification treatment, Kim soon noticed an improvement in her energy and breathing. However, as soon as she ran out of her supplementation, the symptoms would all return. She very clearly needed to change her work environment if we were to make any headway. She was experiencing acute toxic poisoning from chemical exposures. Her body did not have the capacity to cope, and until we could get those exposures elimi-nated, she would continue to deteriorate. It can be a long road to recover from toxic chemical exposure.

Kim's case is a clear example of exposure to acute toxins – however, for most people, toxic exposures are more subtle – low grade and slow to accumulate. As a result, symptoms are generally more vague and insidious than they were with Kim. Whatever the degree of expo-sure, less in and more out is still the motto for any good detox regime. How long that detox process takes to shift symptoms, depends on how many toxins are there, and how much damage there is to repair.

Interesting Facts:

"Of the more than 75,000 chemicals registered with Environmental Protection Agency, only a very small fraction has ever been assessed for their toxicity in humans. In fact, only about 25% of commonly used chemicals have undergone even the most basic toxicity testing."
— *Environmental Defence*[19]

"In Canada, there are over 23,000 chemicals registered for production and use since the 1980s, and up until 2006 the majority had not been rigorously tested for their impacts on human health, or the environment."
— *Environment and Health Canada*[20]

"In 2001 the estimated costs to society suggest that between $568 billion and $793 billion were spent annually in Canada and the US for environmentally-caused disease."
— *Environmental Health Perspectives*[21]

"Studies found levels of about a dozen common organic pollutants to be 2 to 5 times higher inside homes than outside, regardless of whether the homes were located in rural or highly industrial areas. Of these pollutants many are associated with asthma, allergies, nausea, malaise, rashes, lung disease, neurological dysfunction, and even cancer."
— *US Environmental Protection Agency*[22]

Environmental toxins are a very large category to discuss. The fact is that there are not many consumer products that don't contain some form of toxin or another. As discussed at the start of this chapter, by toxin, I am referring to any foreign chemical that alters or affects the body in a negative way. This includes solvents, formaldehyde, drugs, alcohol, pesticides, herbicides, food additives and colourings, preservatives, flavourings, plastics and many more. What makes these substances so damaging on a molecular level is that they mimic our natural hormones, enzymes or nutrients, but do not behave the same way that these natural components do. The mere fact that a toxin has the capability to turn on or off a function in the body, demonstrates that they alter our biochemistry. For example, toxins may turn on an enzyme for longer than necessary, or alternatively, shut it off altogether. The toxin may then create an inflammatory response in the body, to which a system has to respond. Many areas of the body may be affected, depending on what function the toxin is mimicking.

We can classify different toxins by how they behave in the body. Here are the different categories:

1. Irritants (allergic reactions or irritant dermatitis). These chemicals cause an inflammatory response on contact, leading to itching and burning skin, redness, pain and swelling. Common substances include soaps, household cleaners (dish soap, all-purpose cleaners, laundry detergents, fabric softeners and dryer sheets), latex, fragrances, makeup and cleansers, and sunscreens.

2. Respiratory irritants. These substances congest and cause damage to the lining of the lungs, which can lead to conditions such as asthma, COPD and lung cancer. Common substances include asbestos, coal dust, paints, cement dust, tobacco smoke, soot, silica dust, engine and diesel exhaust, ammonia (bleach) and chlorine. Many of us may not be surprised by this list because our bodies quickly tell us they are harmful when we breathe them in and start coughing. However, long term exposures at low levels can be just as harmful as one exposure at a high level.

3. Carcinogens. These substances have been deemed carcinogenic (cancer-causing) because they can disrupt cellular metabolism and destroy genetic material. Examples include triclosan (main ingredient in anti-bacterial soap), asbestos, tobacco smoke, crystalline silica (cleaners), DDT (often in foods), several dyes (foods and personal products) and formaldehyde. This is a huge category, as most traditional household and personal products will have one form of carcinogen or another.

4. Enzyme blockers. These toxins bind to and inhibit the action of enzymes in the body. This may be reversible or irreversible. Carbon monoxide poisoning is a notable example.

Many drugs use this mechanism of action: antibiotics like penicillin, heart medications like Ramipril®, and pain prescriptions like Celebrex®. They either force a new action to happen in the body or stop it from doing something unwanted. These are foreign substances that are not part of normal biochemistry or physiology. That is not to say they can't be life-saving, but long term medication use is often missing the mark in discovering the true imbalances, and can even add to the toxic load.

Pesticides are another common source of enzyme blockers, with the most well-known being glyphosate, sold by trade name Roundup®. It works to inhibit protein synthesis, thereby rapidly killing the plant. It is quickly absorbed and transported throughout the plant and soil, thereby contaminating the soils in the area that weeds are being treated. GMO crops, as previously discussed, have been altered to be glyphosate resistant, meaning they can be sprayed with the toxin and not die or be affected by it. Therefore, the plant can be covered in it by the time of consumption. Beyond GMO crops, glyphosate alone has been linked to tumours in rats; however, as these products are patented, little independent research can be done. Another practice that started in the 1980s, called desiccation, is to heavily spray crops (commonly wheat), with glyphosate to speed up harvest in cold and wet climates. This practice has been largely scrutinized, as it contributes to much higher levels of the toxin right before production. In March 2015, the World Health Organization deemed glyphosate as "probably carcinogenic in humans."[23] Glyphosate has been banned by The Netherlands, Malta, Sri Lanka, El Salvador and Argentina, with Sweden, Brazil, and France currently in deliberations. It is reported that there has been approximately 18.9 billion pounds of glyphosate sprayed globally since 1974, with 70% in the last decade.[24]

5. Free radical producers. Free radicals are reactive molecules that are created when molecular bonds are broken. Imagine two people holding hands, who are happy, balanced and stable. Then imagine another man (free radical) comes along, feeling unbalanced, unstable and incomplete, – and rips apart that initial bond between the two people so he can feel complete. He now leaves the first person (molecule) looking to find someone else to balance them. The process repeats, again and again. The free radicals continue to be created and rip apart enzymes, lipids (fats), DNA and proteins in order to try to balance themselves, and in the process, continue to create new free radicals. This creates damage, also known as oxidative stress, in the body.

Free radicals are a big contributor to aging. This is a normal process of cellular metabolism where tissues break down slowly over time (this is why we don't live forever), but it can get sped up with increased exposure to free radicals.

We also naturally create free radicals, aka reactive oxygen species (ROS), for our immune system to kill viruses and bacteria. However, if too many are created, we get damage. ROS are also accelerated by environmental toxins, as well as stress, trauma, infections, injury and excessive exercise. Substances like cigarette smoke, air and industrial pollution, car exhaust, pesticides, radiation, alcohol, charred or deep fried foods, and many drugs (such as chemotherapy) are common free radical creators in our environment. In fact, the way that chemotherapy works in the body is by causing the same type of damage to the cancer cells. Ironically, free radical damage is linked to the development of all inflammatory diseases, including cancer, heart disease and even sunburn. One of our main defenses against oxidative stress is antioxidants like Vitamin C, Vitamin E, Co-enzyme Q 10, Glutathione and Alpha Lipoic acid (more on treatments in Part 2 of this book).

6. Inflammatory promoters. Inflammation is the body's attempt at self-protection; it attempts to remove harmful substances, including irritants and toxins, in order to support healing. The symptoms of inflammation include pain, redness and swelling. A certain amount of inflammation is good, as it initiates the body to handle and remove any negative substances. However, chronic irritation leads to chronic inflammation and ongoing symptoms. Substances include phthalates, dust, mold spores, tobacco smoke, heavy metals and pollution.

7. Blockers of natural absorption of vitamins, fats and minerals. Common substances include heavy metals, fluoride and various processed foods. They bind to and compete with transport proteins, thereby reducing our ability to absorb essential nutrients. In the case of fluoride, since it has a similar molecular structure to chlorine and iodine, it often blocks the enzymes that require these key nutrients to function. This is a big reason why I always suggest that anyone with thyroid issues (requiring functioning iodine), should be avoiding competing fluoride exposures, often found in drinking water, toothpaste and dental treatments. This may mean filtering water if applicable, using xylitol toothpaste rather than fluoride, and talking to your dentist about your individual necessity for in-office fluoride treatments.

Lead and cadmium are known to affect the absorption of iron, zinc and copper. Anemia is a common issue that affects a large percentage of our population, from infants to the elderly. Could one factor in this deficiency be lead exposure (most likely found in tap water – see following section on heavy metals), rather than simply not getting enough iron? The absorption blocking problems can also be compounded by a lack of quality food in our diets, and an increased requirement in our body, as previously discussed in nutrient deficiencies.

8. Neurodevelopmental disruptors. These toxins are being linked to disabilities in the development of children's brains. This includes Autism, ADHD, dyslexia, delayed development and poor school performance. Drs Philippe Grandjean and Philip Landrigan published a review in The Lancet Neurology in 2014 which found several toxins to be of urgent concern for developmental disabilities. They are urging a dramatic reform in the use and regulation of toxins. They describe the need to regulate these chemicals as an inherent necessity to "control the global pandemic of developmental neurotoxicity." They ascertain that "assessment of toxicity must be followed by governmental regulation and market intervention. Voluntary controls seem to be of little value." They also urge that "these new approaches must reverse the dangerous presumption that new chemicals and technologies are safe until proven otherwise."

Neurodevelopmental disruptors include:

- Lead (shown to affect IQ)

- Methylmercury (found to affect fetus brain development)
- Arsenic (reduced brain function in several studies)
- Toluene (shown to be linked to ADHD)
- Polychlorinated biphenyls or PCBs (reduced cognitive function in young children)
- Manganese (decreased intelligence and ADHD)
- Fluoride (seven point decrease in IQ in children)
- Chlorpyrifos and DDT (physical and neurodevelopmental problems in young children)
- Tetrachloroethylene (hyperactivity and aggression linked)
- The polybrominateddiphenyl ethers (associated with neurodevelopmental problems)
- Bisphenol A (hormone disruptors)
- Phthalates: (reduced attention span)[25]

9. Endocrine and reproductive disruptors. These toxins compete with and/or influence the hormonal functions of our bodies. These include thyroid, brain, adrenal (stress) and male/female hormones. They are often linked to all too common conditions like breast or prostate cancers, infertility, brain function abnormalities and hypothyroidism. Bisphenol A, found in plastics, has been a notorious culprit in the last several years. These hormone disruptors have also been associated with early puberty in girls and childhood obesity.

10. Uncouplers. These toxins affect mitochondrial function, (aka those cellular energy factories, as explained in my Genetics chapter) resulting in accelerated aging and degeneration of body tissues. Nearly every action in a cell requires energy in the form of ATP, which is what your mitochondria produce. Toxins that break that chain of energy production impede your cells' ability to work properly – to absorb nutrients, clear waste, produce proteins, replicate genetic material and so on. Many conditions today are being associated with mitochondrial diseases, where any of your cells could stop producing energy efficiently. Heavy metals are common culprits.

In Kim's case, when she was able to help her system clear the toxins, and even more importantly, remove the acute toxic exposures at work and at home, her symptoms improved. But what about when toxicity is not from current exposures, but rather from low grade and chronic exposures over a longer period of time?

By the time I saw 39-year-old Joyce, she felt she was in a constant state of inflammation. She was developing psoriasis on her scalp and chest. She was extremely fatigued, had poor circulation, hot flashes at night, periodic skin rashes that would break out all over her body, and was highly sensitive to any chemical she was exposed to. She would get an instant headache, dizziness, sinus congestion and nausea when she would stand too close to someone with perfume on, or walk down the cleaning aisle at the supermarket. She couldn't tolerate alcohol at all, and often felt hung over in the morning, even when she didn't drink anything.

Upon review, she didn't report being exposed to any chemicals recently, outside of living close to an apple orchard. She was trying to eat organic and gluten free as much as possible, as she noted this did help her. She lived in a relatively newer townhouse, and worked mostly from home. However, she did grow up in a community with a local mill, she had second hand smoke exposure, growing up with a father who was a smoker, and she drank well water in her childhood as well. She also previously worked in a hair salon for about ten years, and got her nails done monthly for years. She quit hairdressing due to allergy symptoms, especially when she was working with hair dyes, and stopped getting her nail treatments when she kept getting periodic rashes on her hands.

It is key that we understand the overwhelming truth – we are surrounded by environmental chemicals, and we must come to terms with the need to take action to stay healthy. The organic, chemical conscious trend is not just a fad, it is a necessity. With awareness, we can invoke change on a grand scale. You vote with your dollars, so the more you are conscious about what you buy, the more pressure manufacturers and food producers will feel to create safer products. They create the supply where the demand is. Believe it or not, you can make a difference.

Here are some top toxins to look for when shopping:

1. **Bisphenol A:** plastic #7, lining of metal cans, plastic wrap, bottles
2. **Dioxins:** industry, foods (fish, dairy, meats – 90% of human exposure)
3. **Flame retardants:** children's clothing, polyesters, mattresses
4. **Formaldehyde:** cosmetics, glues, paints
5. **Parabens:** cosmetics and personal hygiene products (e.g. soaps, shampoos)
6. **PERCs:** dry cleaning, shoe polish
7. **Pesticides (Organophosphates):** bug sprays, lawn and crop control
8. **Phthalates:** perfumes and scented products, plastic softening (e.g. plastic wrap), food (main source – easily released in environment)
9. **PVCs:** vinyl, hard plastic #3
10. **Triclosan:** anti-bacterial soaps
11. **VOCs (toluene, benzene):** paints, household products, adhesives
12. **Toluene:** solvent in paints, glues, disinfectants, lacquers, fuels
13. **Polychlorinated biphenyls or PCBs:** foods and fish (commonly building up in the environment), coolants, lubricants
14. **Fluoride:** drinking water, toothpaste (especially when swallowed), dental procedures – trace amounts in teeth and bone are required, but damaging in excess
15. **Chlorpyrifos and DDT:** pesticides (banned in the US and Canada but used worldwide in lower income countries)
16. **Tetrachloroethylene:** medical, cleaning, cosmetic career exposures (e.g. nurses, chemists, custodians, hairstylists, beauticians)
17. **Polybrominateddiphenyl ethers:** fire retardants (e.g. in children's clothing, mattresses, couches, carpets)

Also concerning is the fact that many of these toxins are persistent in the environment. As they are not easily broken down, they remain toxic to our earth for a very long time – many taking years to decades to decompose. As we continue to use these substances, they accumulate in the environment at higher and higher levels, making our exposures to them more problematic. They are persistent in our bodies as well. We will attempt to get rid of them if possible, but if not, our body will store them somewhere where they are less harmful. Many toxins can be very difficult to metabolize or break down, so the latter option of storage is all the body can do. This process is called *bioaccumulation*. Substances like heavy metals, PCBs, DDT and pesticides will accumulate in our bodies. They then continue to increase in concentration in the tissues of a living organism throughout its lifetime.

We tend to stuff these harmful substances in our fat and bones because those tissues are more metabolically stable. Our bodies only have a 10% annual turnover of fat and bone cells.[26] Compare this to stomach cells, with a two to nine day turn over, or lung alveoli, which are replaced every eight days. Our bodies are trying to protect us the best way they can – by storing the toxins in areas that will allow for less mobilization. The last thing our bodies want are free floating toxins wreaking havoc in the blood stream. This is why toxins of heavy metals rarely show up in a blood test unless the person had a recent high exposure. Logically then, it makes sense that people often feel sluggish and toxic during a weight loss regime. What is the first thing we will release with fat loss? Toxins! A good weight management regime will always have a detox component to it. We will discuss the process of detoxing in Part 2 of this book.

In Joyce's case, the diagnosis of Multiple Chemical Sensitivities explained the progressive inflammation in her body and may have even contributed to the recent diagnosis of an autoimmune disease psoriasis. She had expressed that she didn't like the idea of taking more medications, as per her current doctor's recent suggestion, so she had sought out other options. Her friend had recommended a cleanse, so she had tried one on her own, only to feel absolutely awful! She instinctively had the right idea – however, in her case, this process

needed to be done very gently. Based on her history of a substantial accumu-
lated chemical toxicity, I determined that her increased burden had led to
more than her body could handle, thus bioaccumulation had occurred.

A cleanse really is defined by bringing less toxins into the body and
moving more toxins out. I use the analogy of a cleanse being like a big
spring cleaning – a deep sanitation of our internal house, so to speak.
However, as mentioned above, most toxins do not reside floating
around in the body (i.e. in our extracellular fluids), yet many cleanses
focus just on that. This inherently can be a bit more aggressive in that
we are mobilizing and moving toxins out of the body from the blood,
lymph and connective tissues. In our house cleaning analogy, it's like
taking the biggest broom you can find and sweeping up all the mess
into a huge pile – choking and gasping at the dust and debris flying
around along the way – until we thrust the door open and everything
flies out on the lawn. No wonder Joyce's already overloaded system
felt awful from a cleanse! Cleanses often include things like milk thistle, infrared saunas, fasting or colonics. Providing the house isn't too
dirty or we clean it regularly, these can be effective and not harmful to
the body.

In Joyce's case, as she was already not coping well with the toxins that were
circulating in her system, she needed an avenue to get them out of the body
before she could even think about mobilizing the stored toxins in her fat and
bone tissues. For her, we used drainage, aka homotoxicology, rather than a
traditional detox. Remember our house analogy? In drainage homotoxicol-
ogy, imagine we sweep all that dust into garbage bags, one by one, first in the
rooms and halls, then in closets, the attic, and the cupboards...we then open
the doors and windows, let the fresh air in, and quietly remove the bags of
filth. This is what Joyce needed – a slow and steady process to gently clear the
toxic burden from her system, without causing further inflammation and
damage in the process. For her, this was a very slow and intentional process
over many months, but it allowed her symptoms to slowly start to improve –
first her headaches and fatigue, and gradually the sensitivity to environ-
mental elements. The psoriasis stopped spreading, but it will be the slowest to
recover – for it is an indication of the degree of dysfunction created by the

toxicity leading to confusion in her immune system. However, eventually this too can shift.

It doesn't appear that the use of toxic chemicals, additives or products will be restricted in their use or production any time soon. In fact, it seems more apparent that newer substances will be added to the mix. Unfortunately, very few of these toxins have substantial studies that are adequate enough to guarantee them safe to the public and the environment. We all seem to be part of a grand experiment – making it that much more important to be our own advocates and seek out better, cleaner options. Part of the courageous cure for your health issues is to learn about how interconnected we are to our environment – and to then realize that we can advocate and choose to make healthier choices not only for ourselves, but also for our planet. The earth is the very thing that sustains us in all of our capacities. So, while the sheer number of toxins can be overwhelming, know that it starts with a positive intuitive choice each and every day. Big global change never happens overnight, but we have the power to be a part of the solution, not the problem.

3) HEAVY METALS

Tom, who was in his mid-40s, came into my office with concerns of chronic itchy skin and jock itch. He was noticing intense itchy rashes on his groin, feet and scalp that simply wouldn't go away. Any creams he tried only gave temporary relief, and it was driving him crazy. It seemed to be spreading, not getting better. Upon investigation, he also reported suffering from some occasional heartburn and indigestion. He lived a busy, active life, but loved his social beer a couple nights a week. He also had a mouth full of mercury amalgams that he had since his teens. To me, there was no question that he was fighting chronic yeast and a fungus called tinea. We started a candida diet, which primarily eliminates sugars, starches and yeast fermented foods, along with adding some yeast killers like grapefruit seed extract and P'au D'arco. He immediately saw improvement, but the problem was that he could never cheat on the diet or stop his supplements, or he would immediately see a flare-up with symptoms. Once we got the infection under control, we could finally uncover the deeper root cause of the itch and unease – he had an excessive chronic heavy metal burden.

Truth is, I have several patients that fit this profile – not just men, but women too –women who have been suffering from chronic vaginal yeast infections, having to take an oral or vaginal anti-yeast treatment month after month, only to find temporary relief. The constant vaginal itching and burning can make intercourse out of the question, because of a deep burning sensation. As in Tom's chronic infection case, the symptoms were resolved with a candida diet and some anti-fungal herbs, but no one should have to be on a candida diet forever! Sure enough, with these patients as well, when we investigated heavy metals and reduced their toxic burden, the yeast cleared up and they could resume a normal healthy diet.

Contrary to what most people think, heavy metals are all around us. They're not just associated with the mercury amalgams in our teeth and lead paints, though these are serious sources. They are found everywhere – in the food we eat, the air we breathe and the things we use. I often tell my patients it's not a matter of *if* heavy metals are present in your body but rather *how much* – and how much are they affecting you?

From a toxicity perspective, there aren't acceptable limits for heavy metals. In fact, no amount of heavy metals are good for the body; they are always damaging, some are just worse than others. However, the problem with traditional blood testing is that it only measures acute exposures, like an industrial spill for example. If a blood lab detects heavy metals in a sample, it will be severely problematic for your health. If you look up the toxicity reports for most heavy metals, you will see descriptions of severe neurological and cognitive problems – from psychosis, to pain, to significant organ impairment. Fortunately, we rarely see acute toxic exposures, but this leaves heavy metals largely underestimated, and often not even considered, in a person's pathology. What's clinically more evident is chronic exposure due to one or more metals in our environment. This is a widespread problem, because our bodies have a very difficult time eliminating heavy metals. Rather, we tend to stuff them away in our fat and bone tissue (much like the environmental toxins). This protects the body from accumulating heavy metals in the blood stream and causing cellular damage, as seen in acute toxicity. However, overtime the can be slowly mobilized or tissue levels can become saturated, leading to chronic low grade exposure.

We are all exposed to heavy metals. Here are some of the most common metals and their most frequent sources:

1. **Aluminum**: COOKWARE, VACCINES, composite dental fillings, cans, aluminum foils, pipes, white flour, deodorant, lipstick.
2. **Antimony**: FIRE RETARDANTS (particularly in children's clothing, mattresses, and other fabric furniture), car batteries, plastics, paint, adhesives, fertilizers, cigarette papers, glass, alloy production
3. **Arsenic**: CIGARETTE SMOKING, soils, emissions (e.g. power plants/smog/smoke), wood preservatives/pressure treated wood, insecticides (especially for ants), shellfish, volcanoes, electroplating, well water, copper mines
4. **Beryllium**: occupational exposure
5. **Bismuth**: Pepto-Bismol®, cosmetics with shimmery metallic finish
6. **Cadmium**: CIGARETTE SMOKING, industrial exposures, contaminated shellfish, acidic beverages in contaminated containers, auto exhaust, plastics, wine
7. **Gold**: gold amalgams, osteoarthritis injections
8. **Lead**: DRINKING WATER, leaded gasoline (prior to 1955), cigarette smoking, cosmetics, hair dyes, mother to infant transfer during pregnancy (heavy metals can pass through breast milk), mini-blinds, metal wicked candles, industrial pollution, batteries, canned foods, lead glazed cookware or pottery or glass (especially from developing countries), some

fertilizers, stained glass creation, home remodeling, lead based paints and oil stains, occupational exposure (plumbers, miners, printers, refiners, welders, auto repair, plastic manufacture, battery manufacture, gas station attendants)

9. **Mercury**: DIET (fish and seafood), VACCINES, DENTAL AMALGAMS, gold extraction, skin-lightening creams, some eye drops, petroleum, natural gas, occupational exposure (e.g. miners), fossil fuel combustion, cement production, pesticides

10. **Nickel**: nickel refinery dust, cigarette smoking, hairspray, jewelry, batteries, shampoo, pipes, tap water

11. **Thallium**: soil deposits west of the North American Rocky Mountains (found in water and food grown in contaminated areas)

12. **Uranium**: dust from mines, drinking water, uranium glass dishes

Chronic exposure to metals can affect many areas of the body over time. The metals can mimic our essential minerals due to a similar molecular structure. They are then able to bind to and disrupt the function of the mineral receptor sites. Minerals are essential for all normal enzymatic activity, so this is why the symptoms of heavy metals will often seem vague and insidious, affecting all aspects of the body. However, there are some body systems that are more negatively affected than others from overexposure. The metals also have concerning compound effects, meaning the more metals we are exposed to, the more deleterious effects they have.

Some of the effects of exposure to heavy metals include:

1. **Nephrotoxicity:** various areas of the kidneys are affected. The function of the kidneys is reduced, and/or effect water balance (hypertension) and/or hormone balance are affected.

2. **Neurotoxicity:** dysregulation of neurotransmitters in the brain. Brain injury and death can occur in newborns. As Health Canada states, infants and children are at the highest

risk for this effect.[27] This effect is also linked to neurological conditions like Autism,[28] Parkinson's, and Alzheimer's.[29]

3. **Immunotoxicity**: even at levels considered "non-toxic," heavy metals can suppress immune systems. This causes decreased resistance to bacterial infections, as well as increased susceptibility to viruses, fungi and parasites. Chronic, repetitive infections may occur. Autoimmune disease and cardiovascular disease have also been linked to immunotoxicity.[30]

4. **Allergies**: as the immune system is suppressed, we also develop antigens to heavy metal/protein complexes in the body, leading to chronic allergies. We may also see eczema, psoriasis, scleroderma and other skin conditions associated with this toxic effect.

5. **Hormonal imbalances**: the endocrine system is negatively affected – function of the pituitary gland, thyroid gland, thymus gland, adrenal gland, as well as enzyme production processes are affected, even at very low levels of heavy metal exposure. These disruptions may lead to hypothyroidism, autoimmune disease, infertility, menstrual problems, frequent miscarriages, fibroids, endometriosis, menopausal symptoms and hormonal imbalances.[31]

Specific causal links associated with heavy metals and effects on the body:

1. **Aluminum**: incoordination, poor memory, depression, tremors, impaired cognition, lung and bladder cancer, behaviour difficulties, colic, liver dysfunction, Alzheimer's

2. **Antimony**: respiratory tract problems, cardiac depression, skin problems, menstrual irregularities, miscarriage, weakness, tremors

3. **Arsenic**: skin, liver, lung, kidney and bladder cancer; hormone imbalances, liver deterioration, skin afflictions, gastrointestinal distress, malaise, muscle weakness,

cardiovascular disease, garlic breath, altered sensations of hands and feet

4. **Beryllium**: lung cancer
5. **Bismuth**: stomatitis, increased salivation, pathological fracture (osteoporosis), encephalopathy
6. **Cadmium**: leg cramps, nausea, vomiting, diarrhea, joint pain, kidney stones, yellow teeth, dry skin, hair loss
7. **Gold**: kidney problems
8. **Lead**: fatigue, headaches, poor memory, attention deficit, decreased coordination, peripheral neuropathy (loss of feeling in extremities), anemia, kidney problems, lowered immune system, lowered sperm count, hormonal imbalances, hypertension, permanent reduction in IQ levels in children
9. **Mercury**: irritability, excitability, anxiety, restlessness, depression, insomnia, delirium, kidney toxicity, gastric pain, gingivitis, thyroid problems, neurotoxicity, tremors, autism, negative effects on neurological development in infants
10. **Nickel**: lung and nasal sinus cancer
11. **Uranium**: lung cancer

As we suspected that Tom had been chronically exposed to heavy metals – likely through his amalgams, second hand cigarette smoke as a child, and several other common ways as listed in the chart above – we decided to proceed with a heavy metal test. This urine test gives us the best estimate of which metals are in the system and how much the body has accumulated over a life span. Tom did a urine provocation test to determine his chronic heavy metal body burden. Heavy metal tests must be done with a provoking agent (aka chelating agent) to determine this body load. A chelating agent is a compound that is not metabolized by the body, has high affinity to bind metals, and is eliminated quickly by the body, carrying the metal out with it. If an unprovoked or random test is performed without a chelating agent, whether through urine, hair or even blood, it will only tell us current exposures.

Remember the majority of chronic metals are stored in fat and bone, so we want the test to pull out those "stuffed away" metals so that we can understand the total body burden. Tom's test for metals came back elevated in mercury (ten times the suggested safe level) and lead (five times the suggested safe level). We began a twelve-month process of clearing these metals through EDTA and DMPS IV therapy, and he slowly but surely was able to stop all candida treatments and not have a reoccurring rash or infection. Did I mention his heartburn was also resolved? Fungal infections in the stomach are a big contributing factor to heartburn, indigestion, belching and hiatal hernias! Once the infections were cleared, he could support normal acid and functioning of the stomach.

Determining the heavy metal burden should always be done with an unprovoked test (random urine test) and a provoked test (with a chelating agent for a set time, typically six to ten hours). Since the unprovoked represents current exposures, it is important to have the provoked to represent total body burden. This combination allows us to get the best estimation of what your body has been holding onto, from existing exposures to exposures over your whole lifetime. If you don't do both tests, you may wrongly assume the metal burden is all from old exposures and miss addressing a current source.

Once tested, various chelation techniques can be chosen based on the metals that are present. Ethylenediaminetetraacetic acid (better known as EDTA), typically administered via intravenous, is the father of chelation and is an excellent choice for lead, cadmium, aluminum and arsenic. It is particularity good for pulling lead from the bone (lead's favourite place to be stored). EDTA has also been used traditionally to treat atherosclerosis by clearing plaque build-up in the arteries, but I wonder how much of that damage is from the heavy metals as well?

2,3-Dimercapto-1-propanesulfonic acid (also known as DMPS), also best administered through an IV, is an excellent choice for removing elemental mercury, namely from dental amalgams. I always recommend the amalgams are removed before this method is used, so you're not just pulling the mercury out of your amalgams. The disadvantage of this chelating agent is that it is often the most poorly tolerated, with a small percentage of people having allergic reactions to it due to its rich abundance of sulphur molecules.

Lastly, Dimercaptosuccinic acid (also known as DMSA), the one oral chelation method, is more of a broad spectrum chelator. Some people debate whether this is a true chelating agent, but I have found it effective for covering the removal of a large variety of metals for patients at a more affordable cost. The drawback to this chelating agent is its potential for redistribution. Because it attracts more types of metals like lead, methylmercury (found in fish and the environment) and uranium, it doesn't bind to the metals as tightly. For example, when DMSA binds to a metal (e.g. lead) in one area of the body (e.g. the brain) and then works its way through the system, it can be detached from the chelating agent by something else, possibly even a mineral like magnesium. This causes the metal to redistribute from one area of the body (brain) to another (say muscle), often causing inflammatory symptoms. I believe this is one of the unfortunate realities of this method – symptoms like headaches, fatigue and nausea are often reported by patients using DMSA. When administered properly – meaning the correct dose, break times in between administration, and supportive supplements – the symptoms from the chelating agents can be very minimal and treatment is very successful.

Chelation should always be done under the supervision of a certified physician. It's important to know the strengths and limitations of each of the methods so that you can make the most informed decision on how to proceed. Chelation, although a slow process, can be life changing for people who have suffered from chronic disease. I have used chelation to successfully treat infertility, Lyme disease, chronic yeast, tumour growth, MS, urticaria, gout and heart disease, just to name a few.

A Note on Vaccinations:

For the purpose of this book, I'm not going to discuss the merits of vaccination, as there has been evidence over the years that does support the use of vaccines for some endemic infections. Hence this section is not advice on whether or not to vaccinate. In fact, my college regulatory body, supports the current vaccination model with adequate education for the patient. Yet is it still hotly debated even within my own profession. But despite the debate, I do believe that most people see the value and merit of the discovery of vaccines. Smallpox was the first infection to use a vaccine-like method, and it has been eradicated from our world population since 1978. Polio is another illness that has been drastically reduced. I would say there is conclusive evidence that supports that at least for the short term, many vaccines do work to prevent or lesson the severity of infections.

I refer to the evidence as short term, because vaccines do not support lifetime immunity development for the majority of infections – hence why boosters are required. How "immunity" is defined is debated as well, as the presence of antibody titers in the blood may, in fact, not dictate immunity for all vaccines.[32] There are still many unknowns around the effects of vaccines. We do know that herd immunity – the more people with the vaccine, the greater reduction in the spread of infection – is effective for some infections, like Rubella, though this is not a universal principle for all infections, for example, Tetanus.

I will discuss the potential long term concerns based on the nature of vaccines and their components from a toxicity standpoint, as I don't believe these have been sufficiently investigated. Just taking a quick look at the immediate outcomes without taking into account the risks associated with the vaccines does not give us the basis for informed decisions. Short term gain versus long term strain is not a very good formula to be working with, especially if the infections we are talking about (the flu for example), are neither severe nor life threatening for the majority of the population.

There are two points of consideration I want to cover in this chapter of the book:

1. Toxic additives that are required in the making of vaccines are a concern for many people. These components allow for the creation, stabilization and effectiveness of the vaccine. However, these additives are injected directly into the body, out of range of where our immune defenses are normally concentrated. Toxins usually enter through the digestive tract, the lungs or the skin, where our immune system is set up to deal with these exposures more optimally.

Common toxins in vaccines include:

*   the heavy metal mercury aka thimerosal (primarily today just in the flu vaccine and Hep B in Canada)
*   the heavy metal aluminum (in all vaccines)
*   the antibiotic neomycin (or other antibiotic derivative in all vaccines)
*   yeast
*   the preservative formaldehyde

- growth mediums (sourced from a variety of animal cells such as chicken embryo, monkey's kidney, mouse brains, duplicated human cells [HeLa cells], diploid cells [aborted fetus cells], among others)

Another issue with these added toxins is that they are injected into the body several times over! Every time a vaccine is given, these components are also included. It has been deemed medically necessary to administer multiple doses over time for most vaccines, in order for the vaccine to be considered statistically effective for the majority of the population. It has not been established what amount of exposure to these toxins a little body can handle. What is the cumulative effect of the toxins from several different vaccinations over a long period of time? Most of the research is controversial, is often biased, and concludes with weak evidence that neither confirms nor denies health problems may be caused by vaccinations.[33][34] The long term implications are really not fully studied.

Also problematic, infants' and toddlers' tiny little bodies do not have nearly the same detox capacity nor space to distribute toxins as adults' bodies do. Where there have been links made to health issues, the studies have later been retracted after much controversial attention.[35] Most vaccination studies primarily focus on the immediate (first thirty days) response to a vaccine. The studies look for possible toxicity side effects like developmental disorders or "vaccine injuries," as published in the Vaccine Injury Table. However, if these effects take months or even years to develop, there will be little ability to make an effective correlation to the vaccine. Thus the problem would more likely be seen to be one of many contributing factors, so the sole liability could not be given to vaccines by themselves, which, for all intents and purposes (as I hope you are learning in this book), very well may be the case.

So as we examine this issue (and other issues around toxicity), we have to think about – of the many toxins that we *can* control, which ones do we want to choose to avoid? Consider – do we need more research about the long term toxicity of vaccines versus the efficacy? Are there safer forms and ingredients that we can use instead? I can't answer these questions for you, though I believe if we are looking at all the angles, asking the right questions, and performing unbiased effective studies, we can all feel more confident about our decisions.

2. The second consideration around the safety of vaccinations that I want to discuss in this book is the long term effect of vaccines on the immune system. The information on this topic has been investigated thoroughly by Dr. Tetyana Obukhanych, author of the book *Vaccine Illusion*, with post-doctoral work at both Stanford University and Harvard Medical School. In an interview with Catherine J. Frompovich, she discussed concerns around contamination of the growth mediums in vaccines – that they have "the potential to result in sensitization to these proteins or even to break human immunologic tolerance to 'self.' The latter is especially relevant to infants, since their immune system is only starting to make the distinction between 'self' and 'foreign.' Setting this distinction the wrong way from the start, in my view, is likely to pave the road to allergic or autoimmune

manifestations." So the concern is, if we continue to expose our bodies to components in vaccines, what are we doing to the *function* of our immune systems long term? Are we pushing that immune system to become confused or imbalanced? Will we start creating reactions or antibodies to more innocuous foods or environmental substances because of this imbalance? So many things are unclear. The study of immunology is actually a barrier to finding the answers to these questions. This sole area of study was only created when vaccines were invented to determine how these "foreign" components react in the immune system, not how the immune system actually works!

What is clear is that the majority of all vaccines themselves do not impart lifetime immunity to an infection the way our innate immune system would. As Dr. Obukhanych further comments in her interview, this means a "vaccination does not engage the genuine mechanism of immunity. Vaccination typically engages the immune response – that is, everything that immunologists would theoretically 'want' to see being engaged in the immune system. But apparently this is not enough to confer robust protection that matches natural immunity." [36]

I believe we need to learn much more about the long term consequences of vaccines. Would it be more effective to support our immune systems or develop ways to help the body fight infections once exposed – so that our long term, naturally developed immunity that has been with us since the dawn of time has a fighting chance? Or is there a less toxic way to apply vaccination technology, as it is clear vaccines have made historical leaps in the fight of infectious deleterious diseases? What do you think?

Summary

Whew, we made it through that chapter! It is heavy, no pun intended. I put a lot of information in this chapter – not to overwhelm you, but to provide you with ample fuel to quench your thirst for knowledge about toxins! Here is the bottom line of what you need to know:

1. Toxins are everywhere! The reality of our world dictates we can't escape them, so if you think they aren't a problem for you, think again!
2. Toxins enter our body through the food we eat, the air we breathe and substances we absorb.
3. The liver, lungs, colon, kidneys, skin and lymphatics system do the bulk of the work in processing and eliminating toxins,

but often our toxic exposures go beyond what the body can handle.

4. There are three main sources of toxins: food, environmental and heavy metals. We are required to make informed decisions to avoid them as much as we possibly can.

The fight against toxicity really comes down to using our consumer power to make more informed choices. Be aware of what you buy and where it comes from. Inevitably, if we pollute, contaminate, strip and destroy our environment, it will no longer provide the safe, viable elements that we need to sustain life. Dealing with toxicity is just as much an environmental issue as it is a health issue. Take care of the world, so it can take care of you.

FOUR

Infections
_____

"The microbe is nothing; the terrain is everything."
~ *Claude Bernard, recounted and confirmed by Louis Pasteur, the father of the Germ Theory.*

ACUTE INFECTIONS

When I discuss infections in this chapter, I am primarily going to discuss the issue of chronic infections, as opposed to acute, as it applies to chronic illness. Typically, infections affect our bodies acutely, and if our immune system is balanced, we will inherently be able to clear them. We are not a sterile organism, we are literally bathing in microbes all the time. Our human cells are outnumbered by microorganisms by a ratio of 10:1! Wow, for every cell we have, there are ten more foreign microflora. This means that naturally we are bombarded with all sorts of microorganisms all the time: some beneficial, some harmful. This is called the microbiome.

The ebb and flow of your flora balance can determine the difference between whether or not you catch the flu. Many of the organisms in us are opportunistic, which means they will only thrive in you, the host, at taxing numbers if the conditions are right. What conditions, you might ask? Well, whether your nutrient intake is optimized, your flora balance is healthy and strong, your immune system function is complete, or if toxins or any other damaging agent that may throw your system off are present. Many of us know that when we are "run down" from too much stress, travel or too many sleepless nights, we ultimately feel more vulnerable to infections.

On a larger scale, our exposure to microorganisms has never really changed over generations. Immunology would suggest that we are exposed to pathogens to help develop and strengthen our immunity. We have normal exposures to organisms that teach and develop our immune system over our life span. These exposures play a large part in developing resilience and resistance to unwanted organisms. A perfect example is developing what's known as dysentery or travelers' diarrhea when traveling to a foreign country. The local population is unaffected because the organisms causing the dysentery are already a part of their normal gut flora, so they have already created resistance to infection. However, as the foreigner has different gut microbes, they are susceptible. The microorganisms occurring in our gut flora vary according to region. Where you live, the food you eat, the climate you live in, and the environmental exposures you have largely determine your microbiome.

So, if infections are part of a normal, healthy immune development, why is it then that we are seeing more and more reoccurring infections, dormant infections, repetitive infections and finally latent infections? The answer lies in the functioning of the immune system.

Infections will take the opportunity to thrive in a weakened immune system, leading to further inflammation and damage. Damage could be caused by many factors. For example, did you know that we all have C. difficile in our digestive tracts, and that this bacteria only becomes a problem if it overgrows, usually through the use of an antibiotic that wipes out other gut flora?

While my focus in this chapter is on the role of infections as an important root to disease, I also want people to understand that if chronic infections are present, something is compromising the immune system. I believe that our immune systems were inherently created to be able to detect and fight "bugs" with stealth and rigour. However, over the years, I and many of my colleagues are seeing a general trend towards an increased amount of infections, more persistent infections, and infectious illnesses that are more difficult to clear from the body. I am convinced that bugs are not getting more and more virulent (or harmful), but rather our immune systems are getting more and more run down.

What does all this mean? The microflora that make up our micro-biome or "terrain" naturally live in us and on us, so they are the key to our survival and immune health. Therefore, the presence of an infection shows us that there was likely a prior flora imbalance. Since, as mentioned above, our human cells are outnumbered by microbes by 10:1, it's no wonder these microbes can have such a huge influence on our overall health, for good and for bad. Keeping our terrain healthy and strong is what prevents these infections from colonizing and taking over. So as we learn about infections in this chapter, please keep in mind – as important as it is to identify and appropriately address an infection, it is equally important that we deal with the underlying root causes (toxins, nutrient deficiencies, etc.) that is compromising the microbiome to result in an infection in the first place.

CHRONIC INFECTIONS

When nineteen-year-old Tory came to see me, she was getting strep throat infections several times a year. She had recently gotten over yet another infection with a strong load of antibiotics. She was in university, and found she was having a hard time keeping up with her busy schedule. She had been having repetitive infections since she was about fourteen years of age, with infections occurring every three or four months. She also reported having several ear infections as a child, and frequent gas, bloating and constipation for as long as she could remember. She seemed to need a lot of sleep and her energy was generally low.

When I examined her tonsils, they were as big as walnuts. They also had tiny crypts in them (pockets that accumulate food and bacteria and lead to tonsil stones) resulting in bad breath that she couldn't ever resolve despite endless dental hygiene efforts. Although her tonsils weren't acutely infected at the time, I could see she had some significant scar tissue in her tonsils. She said the size of her tonsils never seemed to reduce, but it didn't bother her that much unless she had an acute strep infection.

I knew there was likely some biofilm and latent infection in her tonsils, as this is often where infections like strep like to hang out in waiting. The infection would lie dormant just waiting until she would get a little run down – from increased stress or a viral infection, for example.

We started treatment in Tory's case by working on digestive health, as her immune system would never fight infections if it was always challenged with inflammation. We tested for IgG food allergies, which showed a reaction to dairy and sugar, and worked on eliminations. I also started her on a yeast clearing protocol as there were signs of a large overgrowth due to the repetitive antibiotic use.

Fairly quickly her digestion and energy improved, yet the size of her tonsils and resulting susceptibility to strep throat still needed to be resolved. We started some neural therapy on her tonsils, an injection technique that effectively brings blood flow and healing to an area, and breaks down scar tissue. I also started her on some antibacterial herbs, because I knew there was a good chance that when we opened up the biofilm or scar tissue in her tonsils, she would develop another strep infection. We needed to be ready. She did get a slight sore throat after the treatment, but it didn't develop into a full blown strep infection. This was the first time in years this symptom didn't result in infection. With additional scar tissue treatment and continued antibacterial therapy, her tonsil size was halved within a few weeks! We did two more neural therapy treatments, and her tonsils continued to shrink in size with no further infection. We followed up with gut healing remedies and probiotics to once more restore her healthy flora.

Now, several years later, although she has had a few colds and flus since, she has never developed another strep throat infection. She continues to avoid dairy, and her bowels and digestion have never been better.

Chronic infections occur because they are not fully cleared from the body. They slowly and steadily cause inflammation and damage to the system, often over a long period of time. They may also be latent, waiting in hiding to come out at a more opportune time, like shingles. Chronic infections may be parasitic, fungal, bacterial or viral. Any of these infections can take advantage of a weakened immune system and further the immune imbalance thereby increasing inflammatory damage.

I have seen chronic infections as a root cause of disease time and time again in my practice. I believe I first came to understand this reality ten years ago when I started studying and learning about Lyme disease. Lyme disease consists of a collection of various bacteria, predominantly Borrelia burgdorferi, but may also include concurrent infections like Bartonella, Babesia, Erlichia, Rickettsia or Mycoplasma, to name a few. Lyme may also include other types of organisms like parasites or viruses. In chronic or latent Lyme disease, the bacterial infections go largely undetected by the immune system, wreaking havoc on several systems – prominently the musculoskeletal and neurological systems. Significant clinical symptoms that always makes me suspect Lyme associated infections is chronic pain of some sort – for example, headaches, or pains in the joints or muscles – paired with some sort of neurological symptom such as numbness, shooting pains, altered sensations, weakness or an impact on cognitive function (like brain fog, confusion, poor memory or even seizures). These symptoms often take months to years to become apparent and disabling, which I believe leads to infections often being overlooked.

Conventional doctors have been historically used to thinking about infections in terms of acute illnesses like strep throat, urinary tract infection, or even meningitis or septicaemia - infections that may become life threatening. Yet, I would venture to say that inflammatory illnesses, often assumed to have unknown causes, are far more often caused by infections. I believe the huge category of "autoimmune disease" falls into this category. Any chronic inflammation always makes me wary of infections. Lyme is an example of just one type of infection a person may be exposed to. However, as I was learning and treating Lyme, I quickly discovered any infection can become chronic *if* the body allows it, bacteria or otherwise.

Before we dive into discussing the effects of these many types of infections themselves, we will first learn exactly how infections can become chronic.

Chronic Infection Development

There are a few different ways chronic infections develop:

1. Imbalanced Acquired Immunity (TH1/TH2)

Our immune system is a very complex dynamic system – that we are learning more and more about each and every day. For the purpose of this book, I'm going to describe it in a simplistic form, but know that it is much more intricate. In general, our immune system has two pathways. The first pathway we are born with – Innate Immunity. It is our first line of defense and includes cells like Phagocytes and Natural Killer Cells, which detect and destroy abnormal cells and microbes. For the most part, we never know the innate pathway is working because it is so tightly regulated that it has minimal associated generalized symptoms.

However, if our innate pathway is unable to fully do the job of defending our immune system from attackers, we then rely on our Acquired Immunity – the second immune pathway that we continue to develop throughout our lifetimes from all of our microbial exposures. It is where we harness specific microbial attacks and memory of infections. The acquired immune system additionally has two sides to it – Cell-mediated Immunity (also generally known as TH1) and Humoral Immunity (also generally known as TH2). (*See diagram.*)

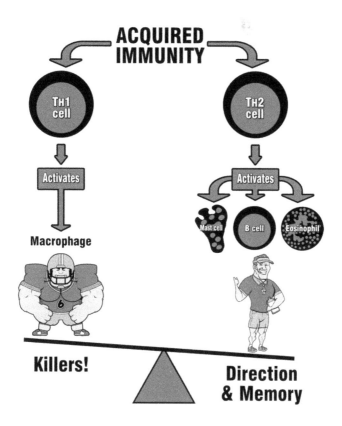

TH1 in our acquired immunity, the cell-mediated immunity, is the killing force. This is where we find white blood cells called Neutrophils and Macrophages. These large cells engulf and remove specific infections or abnormal cells. I often refer to these white blood cells that move through the bloodstream and lymphatic system, as the big football players, working as a team to destroy the opponent.

TH2, the humoral immunity, assists the killers like a coach, marking and directing where the players need to attack. These white blood cells include Basophils, Mast Cells and Eosinophils. This immunity will also provide memory, through antibody production from B cells, so that we never forget all the "plays" on how to beat a particular opponent. And this whole game is orchestrated to make our immune system function in the most efficient way possible.

As long as all players in this system are in balance and working together, the immune system can do its job. However, if any one of our root causes of disease discussed in this book creates an imbalance, then one side of the acquired immunity becomes dominant. As you can see from the diagram above, the two sides need to be in balance, or one will go up and the other will go down, like a teeter-totter.

In the circumstance where the TH2 side becomes more dominant, we get too many coaches directing the plays. When it is chronically imbalanced however, this causes conditions like allergies, asthma, arthritis, eczema or even cancer. This TH2 dominance (increase) causes a release of cell signalers called cytokines, which thereby suppress our TH1 or killer cells (decrease). (See diagram below). We get lots of flagging and direction, but inefficient attacking and killing. Hence, we get a lot of marking and inflammation along with poor infection and tumour cell clearing. TH2 is responsible for creating histamine, so it's dominance will lead to the body making either an allergic or inflammatory reaction. Any "itis" disease we can name is related... gastritis, dermatitis, tendonitis, etc.[38]

TH2 Dominance

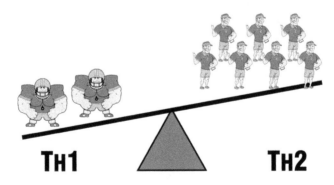

TH1   TH2

On the contrary, if the TH1 side becomes more dominant, we tend to see more killing of infectious and abnormal cells, but less efficiency. This loss in accuracy can lead to substantial collateral damage. The increase in attackers causes destruction to the body, which is related to several autoimmune disorders – including MS, Crohn's or Parkinson's.[39] (*See diagram.*)

TH1 Dominance

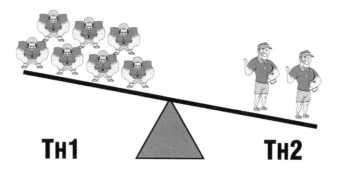

TH1   **TH2**

Interestingly, chronic infections can not only be attributed to an underlying immune imbalance, *but* can also cause the imbalance in the first place! The longer an infection stays in the body, the more it influences that imbalance, just by the nature of the damage and inflammation it causes. This is a big reason why some infections, such as Lyme disease, become persistent, and again brings us to the importance of addressing all the factors or roots influencing immune function when clearing an infection. In Tory's case, described earlier in this chapter, this meant dealing with food allergies, compromised digestive function, other infections, nutrient deficiencies and stress.

1. Persistent exposure:

Another common cause of chronic infections is a persistent exposure. This scenario particularly comes up more often when a person is repetitively being exposed to a toxic pathogen. This could relate to a logical consequence – constantly drinking a contaminated source of water, for example – which naturally will cause a dominance of that organism in the body. However, what I find in clinical practice is unfortunately more often a chronic exposure to organisms such as molds. Black molds especially are very pathogenic. Exposure and infection leads to a constant drain on the immune system, yet often mold is not visually invasive in homes, so people may be unaware of its presence. In the circumstance of mold, typically the respiratory system is affected initially, and people, especially kids, will come into my office with repetitive colds and flus, chronic bronchitis, asthma, allergies, sinus congestion or repetitive ear infections... not to mention fatigue. As the microbe persists in the environment, it continually strains the immune system, since the body is never able to clear it. This can unfortunately open the door to other infections, as the immune resilience is constantly compromised.

2. Root Canals:

Teeth are like any other organ in the body in that they require blood supply, lymphatic drainage and nervous innervation or connection. So, when a tooth becomes infected to the point where the pulp is showing decay, the tooth is considered no longer vital, and is likely to cause continued infection or abscess.

Root canals are often performed in this circumstance, but they ultimately end in a dead tooth being left in the body. This can be a problem, since this dead tooth can result in a breeding ground for infection. Anaerobic (without oxygen) bacteria can thrive in the microtubules of the teeth, an area in your teeth that the dentist is not easily able to get into or clean. Because the root canaled tooth no longer has blood flow or nerve tissue within the tooth, if infection is still present not only will we not feel it, but the body's immune cells are never able to get to the infection within the tooth to fully clear it.

When Jerry came to see me, he was looking for some help with his neuropathy in his toes that he had had ever since his double hip surgery. He had originally had severe osteoarthritis in both hips, but after his surgery the pain was largely resolved. He then developed chronic low back stiffness, difficulty walking and abnormal nerve function. His nerve damage was likely from the surgery, but he reports that it may also have begun before that. We started with some rounds of neural therapy, an injection technique to improve nerve function and increase microcirculation, to try to repair the nerves. We noticed modest improvement.

It wasn't until I was intuitively led to address his dental state that he informed me of a more than twenty-year-old root canal in his front left tooth. He didn't have any pain in it, but I suggested an experiment – treating the root canalled tooth with neural therapy, which could temporarily remove a block, to see if his nerve symptoms improved. By the time he got off the table, without having done any other treatment, the stiffness in his low back was improved and he had increased flexibility. Miraculous! We did the experiment a second time just to be sure. There was no doubt about it, he felt improvement just by addressing the tooth! The problem was, the relief was temporary, because inevitably the tooth interference was still there. He would have to investigate the condition of the root canal.

He tried a local dentist who investigated the tooth but felt there was no issue with the root canal and recommended to leave it alone. I referred him to a trusted biological dentist to have the tooth examined. He had the root canal removed, and upon removal the tissue oozed out pus and smelled putrid. The remaining tooth was literally falling apart. He was amazed at what came out of there! Since then he reports that his feet are much better, he has less stiffness in the back (in fact, it now only occurs in the morning), increased energy, improvement of his constant rhinitis (runny nose), and a stronger resistance to infections. This root canal was there for decades! Who knows what could have been prevented if it had been addressed sooner! I have seen similar stories to Jerry's, where once the person's infected root canals are addressed, their symptoms take a dramatic shift in the right direction. There is no more drain on the immune system.

The constant taxing on the immune system from a latent root canal infection results in the surrounding tissue constantly having to deal with a slew of infectious debris and toxins being created. What's worse, antibacterial treatments, including antibiotics, can't actually penetrate the infection because it's hiding and thriving in the dead, impenetrable tooth. Antibiotics would not be able to be delivered to the infected tooth, it will only ever affect the surrounding tissue and gums. This is why an injection at the tooth site made a notable change for Jerry, as treatment was able to reach the source. Hence, if you have ever had an abscessed root canal in the past, be highly suspicious that the tooth may be chronically infected and weakening your immune system. Even if it hasn't abscessed, it is still important to rule out an underlying infection if you are faced with chronic disease.

Infected root canals have been linked with all sorts of chronic diseases including Lyme disease, autoimmune diseases like inflammatory bowel disease, heart disease and even cancer. For further information on this topic read *The Uninformed Consent* by Dr. Hal Huggins and Dr. Thomas Levy.[40]

An alternative to a root canal is a tooth extraction. Then, depending on the necessity of the tooth for bite and appearance, it can be replaced with a bridge, implant or perhaps in the near future even regrown with the use of stem cells! There currently are studies underway attempting to develop this technique.[41]

3. Biofilms:

Biofilm is not a new concept – however, it is often overlooked when infections are present in the body. A biofilm is a protective matrix that is created around a microorganism when it is threatened. A common example is dental plaque on your teeth, which is formed from bacterial organisms in the mouth. Biofilm is a form of defense – a protein matrix that acts like a cocoon to help the organism survive in less opportune environments. A biofilm can also contain the genetic material from several types of organisms – from parasite, to yeast, bacteria or virus. These organisms are not exactly working together for protection, but they are certainly taking advantage of each other. A common example of this type of symbiotic relationship is seen in nature with pond scum on a water reservoir. Hence, biofilms are a common occurrence by any microrganism, however the type of a biofilm created is what can make them so difficult for your immune system, like scar tissue for example.

Clinically, I commonly see biofilm in the tonsils from repetitive infections like strep throat, as seen in the case study with Tory at the beginning of this chapter. In these cases, the patient often won't have an active acute throat infection, but their tonsils will be full of scar tissue and look to be the size of golf balls! These biofilm scars harbour the dormant microbes, just waiting for the next opportunity to wreak havoc in the system. In this way, repetitive infections are not actually unique each time, but rather the same infection that appears over and over again, as it has just been hiding out in the biofilm.

Biofilms are linked to many repetitive infections such as: bladder infections, vaginal yeast infections, sinusitis and infections related to catheter use and contact lenses to name a few. Atherosclerotic plaque is an associated biofilm, and is a big concern with heart disease and strokes! As any organism can create a biofilm, it is very important that in the treatment of chronic infection, biofilm is also addressed. Biofilms are a big reason why infections may never entirely clear up – remaining at either a low grade level or repetitively flaring up.

If you suffer from a repetitive or chronic infection, definitely suspect biofilm. It most often isn't something you can visually see, so typically must be addressed clinically by doctors at a microscopic level. Because the biofilm is an extracellular protein, remedies that break down protein matrix, like enzymes, are most commonly used in treatment.

4. Polymorphism:

While biofilm refers to the protective matrix organisms can create, another defense micro-organisms can make is change how they look and behave. This is called polymorphism. Polymorphism is the ability of microorganisms to alter their shape or size in response to environmental conditions, like temperature or pH levels. This change in form or "morphology" often causes the immune system to be unable to detect the new form of the altered organism. This phenomenon is common in Lyme disease – when borrelia bacteria is "threatened" by an antimicrobial treatment, it can change its shape into cyst form, thereby evading the specific onslaught of the antibiotic. This is also important to discover in treatment, as different antibiotics will work on different forms of bacteria. Metronidazole antibiotics and grapefruit seed extract are options that fight against cyst forms of bacteria for example.

Parasites

When Heidi came into my office, she was already aware of her persistent parasite, Blastocyst hominis, that she discovered while living part time in Mexico. She had undergone numerous parasite cleanses and prescriptions to try to eradicate the parasite, to no avail. She had been dealing with this parasite for over a year and a half. She was suffering with anxiety, chronic diarrhea, paranoia, nutrient deficiencies and abdominal pain. She was desperate to find answers.

If you are like most people when you hear parasite, you instantly get squeamish. You may have vivid images of revolting worms that are crawling around inside of you. This is where Google is not your friend. Although parasites do include worms, far more of them are microscopic and not even in the digestive tract. They can be in the blood, the lungs, the brain, the skin, the liver, the gallbladder or the lymphatics system, to name a few.

The key here is that parasites by definition are organisms that live in a host (you) and are leaching your nutrients for survival at your expense. They *require* you to live so they are not in the business of destroying you, just stealing from you. Obviously this is still not ideal, but perhaps a more accurate definition that is able to dismantle some of the graphic images from your mind.

Parasites are in fact fairly common. Especially with food handling, parasites can happen anywhere food is manipulated and then not properly cleaned or cooked. Uncooked or undercooked meat, like sushi, can be a common source. It's not just an issue in developing countries, as is often perceived.

We also are a much more global society than in the past, often travelling to various parts of the world several times a year. This exposes us to new or foreign organisms that enjoy making homes in our little host environments.

I discover parasites in my patients all the time, with or without travel. The hardest part to uncovering parasites is that the testing methods we traditionally use are very limited. Unless a parasite is detected on an ova/parasite stool test, the patient is deemed parasite free.

However, what if the parasite isn't in the gut, or it wasn't released at the time of the sample collection? A practitioner can use other private labs to detect parasites, or even use live blood analysis, but unless the parasite is located in the right tissue/blood sample, it simply won't be found.

In my practice I use biofeedback tools in order to understand what the body wants to clear.

> *Biofeedback is a simple tool that relies on the autonomic nervous system to signal a stress reaction to various stimuli in order to give the practitioner insight into what is stressing the body and where it needs support. It is not a diagnostic tool, the way blood tests or X-rays are, nor does it look specifically for abnormalities the way conventional testing does. Biofeedback is looking for imbalances in the system. It can give information around the priority areas for healing, as well as what methods the body will respond to best in treatment. There are many different techniques that can be used in biofeedback: Vega testing, Applied Kinesiology, Autonomic Response testing, EAV, REBA testing, manual muscle testing, bio-resonance, electrodermal testing, BodyTalk, resistance testing and auricular testing, to name a few. Unfortunately, biofeedback techniques have been adopted by too few practitioners. Like many techniques in medicine, the testing is only as good as the tester, so inadequate training and lack of medical intuitiveness can certainly contribute to unreliable testing. These techniques are not new concepts – when properly applied, they can be considered the art of medicine.*

Common symptoms of parasites include:

1. Diarrhea or constipation	2. Abdominal cramps
3. Nausea	4. Fatigue
5. Bloating	6. Skin rashes
7. Mucus in stool	8. Anal itching
9. Teeth grinding	10. Chronic cough and sore throat
11. Allergies	12. Joint pain
13. Malabsorption	14. Night sweats
15. Anemia	16. Dark circles under eyes
17. Pale and/or floating stools	18. Anxiety or restlessness
19. Periodic feeling of malaise	20. Morgellons syndrome

I have also treated many children for parasites, whose number one symptom is temper tantrums with general behavior difficulties. I also commonly see abdominal pain, skin rashes, disturbed sleep, nightmares and teeth grinding. I think this comes up more commonly in children because they are constantly putting their hands and fingers in their mouth and all sorts of place. I can attest to dozens of children over the years who, once on the right remedies, shift their entire demeanor. It's not uncommon for parents to tell me, "I feel like I got my little 'Joe' (or 'Sally') back!"

When the parasite is still physically there, we must address the infection itself with anti-parasitics. Description of these treatments is included in Part 2 of this book under physical healing.

Sometimes the body's immune system is just behaving as if the parasite is there, meaning the immune system is confused. In this case we focus primarily on immune system function, recognizing what it should and shouldn't respond to. Keep in mind, your symptoms are your immune system's reaction to an infection, rather than the infection itself causing symptoms.

This is important to understand as sometimes in my office I may detect infections that are affecting more of the mental and emotional levels rather than just the physical. As you now know, we are outnumbered by organisms 10:1. When our body's cellular balance is skewed by a dominant organism, I do believe it affects many aspects of our lives, including our behavior and emotions. How can you have an emotional parasite, you might say? Well, have you ever been in a parasitic relationship, where you feel like someone is sucking the life out of you? You could call them a parasitic person! I say that half-jokingly, though at times that's what it might feel like. Common parasitic behaviors include narcissism, obsession, negativity, criticism or frustration. You also might sense you are giving away your power too easily by having poor boundaries. You may even experience a "never enough" mentality, feeling like you will never have enough time, energy, support, money, etc. You may feel like you're always running at a deficit and can't catch up.[42] This is where it's important to understand that there are levels to healing, as we will discuss further in Part 2 of this book. Even in the treatment of infections, it may not be just a physical treatment that is required.

Once Heidi was tested in my office using biofeedback, I discovered one of the big reasons she was not clearing her parasite – she was also dealing with a biofilm, that tricky protein matrix that keeps the parasite protected from the immune system. So first we cleared the biofilm with potent enzymes, then we chose an effective remedy and finally started to get things to shift for her. It took four months before she was able to test parasite free in my office and we could start moving into gut repair and healing. After visiting Mexico again the following winter, she repeated the stool analysis for Blastocyst hominis again, just to confirm it was still gone. Not to her surprise, the test came back clear. After her previous struggle for one and a half years of failed treatment with cleanses and prescriptions, she was finally seeing continued healthy digestion. She had regular, normal bowel movements, her energy had returned and she was feeling much more calm and relaxed with the parasite clear.

I often find with infections that if parasites are present, they are the first to show up in the sequence of treatment – largest to smallest so to speak – parasite to fungus to bacteria to virus. They all may be present or there may just be one. Sometimes they may even be inside another infection, like a virus that is contained within a parasite for example.[43]

Determining which we are dealing with comes down to what we've been exposed to – and which related message from our symptoms we need to understand. The mental/emotional picture that these organisms can create could be sending us a message, or vice versa – perhaps we have a susceptibility to those infections because of our predisposition to a similar emotional/mental pattern. Either way, there is a relationship between us and the bug, so we have to change the environment mentally, emotionally, energetically and physically to make it an unfriendly place for that parasite to live. A similar process is needed with other forms of infections. So now let's move down the chain and discuss more around fungal infections.

Fungus

Joanne came to see me in an extremely distressed state. She had a very busy and stressful job which she had always performed quite well, but lately she was really noticing her energy crashing. She was getting sick often, which always seemed to end up in a horrible cough. She also reported having chronic post nasal drip that never seemed to clear, even when she wasn't sick. She had started to notice a wheeze in her breathing when she was active or exercising, yet had no history of asthma. She felt she was reacting to something without a rhyme or a reason, as she was seeing random hive breakouts on her body, which left her feeling confused. Her stomach was off, feeling more bloated and gassy, and overall she just felt run down. As soon as I heard repetitive respiratory infections and sudden onset of a wheeze, I started to suspect a fungal exposure or infection.

A fungus is a type of organism whose purpose is to break down decaying matter and recycle energy in our ecosystems. Therefore, they are abundant and necessary. They play a large factor in the regeneration of forests. Their naturally derived survival mechanisms also provide us with the ability to create antibiotics. Penicillin is made from a fungus! We can never really completely avoid common types of fungi, such as molds and yeast, because they are in us, on us and all around us, all of the time. Yet, they should never be allowed to dominate our flora count. Fungal *infections* originate from a yeast or mold that overgrows in the body.

Fungal organisms are probably structurally the most similar to our human cells. This is one of the reasons anti-fungal medications, like ketoconazole, are often limited in their use, as they can be quite toxic for our body as well.

Although some fungi are toxic, the majority of fungal infections are opportunistic, taking advantage of a system where they are allowed to flourish. For example, the use of antibiotics wipes out normal healthy bacterial flora, literally leaving space for the unaffected fungal bodies to grow unopposed. Antibiotics are a common example, but any root cause that affects our microbiome, like toxins, other infections, stress or GMOs can also lead to this imbalance.

When I see chronic fungal infections in conditions such as irritable bowel syndrome, jock itch, ringworm, chronic sinusitis – or even associated with some types of cardiovascular disease and cancer – I believe we need to take a deeper look at why our body is letting fungi grow.

My first thought in these cases is often to further investigate for heavy metals (mercury specifically) because of their strong correlation to fungal infections. Other factors may also contribute to fungal development, such as food allergies, poor stomach acid, environmental exposures or high chronic dietary exposure to sugars and yeast-containing foods.

Medications like antibiotics or birth control pills, and many toxins are also commonly associated because of the destruction they cause to our healthy flora. Particularly with vaginal yeast, it is also important to treat the woman's sexual partner. Yeast can often be transmitted back and forth, even if the other partner isn't displaying symptoms.

Common symptoms of fungus include:

1. Diarrhea or constipation	2. Bloating and gas
3. Nausea	4. Fatigue
5. Mental fogginess	6. Skin rashes
7. Mucus in stool	8. Muscle and joint pain
9. Craving for sweets	10. Night sweats
11. GERD	12. Obesity
13. Acne	14. Chronic sinus congestion/post nasal drip
15. Vaginal yeast infections	16. Thrush
17. Frequent antibiotic use	18. Athlete's foot, jock itch

I tested Valerie for infections and the first thing to show up was black mold. I asked her very lightly if there was any way that she could be exposed to molds in her home or work environment. She said she wasn't sure, but she had sometimes seen black around her windows. She was living in an apartment building, so didn't have the full background of the building, but did agree that it was an older building. I started some anti-fungal treatment and instructed her to also look for a possible source, since black mold infections typically won't present unless there is some existing in a person's environment. Black mold thrives in warm, damp and humid places, so I had her check her bathrooms, windows and sinks (I'd usually also suggest basements, which wasn't applicable in her case). There was also the unfortunate possibility that airborne spores could be coming through the ventilation system from another apartment and not directly from her own apartment. At her next visit to see me, she revealed that sure enough, not only did she see black mold all around her shower in her poorly ventilated bathroom, but she also discovered it deep in the window frames and even behind the drywall from poorly sealed windows. She was shocked! She unfortunately would have to undergo a full-fledged professional remediation project to ensure her home was not making her sick and was safe to live in.

No wonder Valerie felt run down and tired. It took several months to clear the infection and build up her immune system once she was able to remove herself from her chronic mold exposure. She first had to relocate until the remediation was complete; for as long as she was exposed, her body couldn't make any headway in fighting the fungal infection. When she was away from her apartment, she began to see improvement in her digestive system first, then her energy and mood, and finally her respiratory symptoms. It was a long, uphill battle for her, but a resolution could only be achieved by identifying the persistent source.

Black mold is incredibly toxic. The spores, called mycotoxins, are released and once inhaled, cause damage and a serious immune system threat. If an area smells musty or damp, suspect mold! There are five toxic strains of black mold, including Stachybotrys chartarum, Cladosporium, Fusarium, Penicillium and Aspergillus niger. They don't usually grow in plain sight, so we often have to dig to find them, which can be difficult when they are behind walls or structures. If you suspect mold, however, always hire a remediation company to address the problem. The cleanup process, when you are moving the spores around and releasing the mycotoxins, can be the most toxic. I often have patients tell me they just bleach mold every time it shows up and I want to cry, "Noooo!" For the sake of your health, I urge you to address it properly with expert advice, so that you clear it for good and remedy the reason as to why the mold is there in the first place.

Yeast and molds can affect our emotions as well – OR, perhaps we are susceptible to yeast and molds because of the emotions we are experiencing.[44] Common themes are around self-doubt, inability to trust and irritation. You may also feel scattered, clouded, stressed or stuck. You may feel frustrated with others or yourself. I also often see an association with emotional repression of negative feelings like anger and frustration. As stated in *The Secret Language of your Body* by Inna Segal, you may be "feeling angry that you aren't getting what you want, but not wanting to change or take a positive action (to create it)."[45] This frustration may become apparent during the process of healing and change, but keep in mind, it's necessary to shift to achieve a place of balance. These shifts often come from both conscious and unconscious healing, discussed more in Part 2 of the book.

Often people experience a "die off" with yeast infections (for example, with the "Candida" strain). While the infection has been massively destroyed, collateral damage causes a temporary flare until the body can eliminate the "rubble" left over from the elimination. This is similar to a healing crisis, where sometimes you have to get worse before you can get better. Particularly with yeast, this can bring out feelings of frustration or anger alongside the physical symptoms. It's all just part of the process of clearing infections physically, consciously and unconsciously.

Bacteria

When Susie came into my office, she was in a desperate state. She felt completely at a loss as to why she was experiencing so many disabling symp-

toms. She had always felt she was healthy, so when symptoms of incapaci-
tating fatigue, burning feet, insomnia, night sweats, joint pain and migratory
nerve symptoms started a year earlier, she was left frustrated and confused.
The medical doctors didn't seem to have any answers for her, as all of her
blood work came up normal. I suspected Lyme disease, even though she didn't
report having a bullseye rash or even remember getting bitten by a tick –
which I find very few patients do. We started some antimicrobial treatment
and scheduled an IGeneX® western blot test for six weeks later. In the case of
chronic Lyme, this blood test measures your immune system's antibodies
specifically for the Borrelia bacteria. I always suggest that a patient starts on
treatment six weeks prior to testing because this will help activate the
immune system so we can get a more accurate test result. Initially, Susie
didn't feel well on the antimicrobial treatment, which was further confirma-
tion that an infection was being killed off, so we weren't surprised when her
test results were positive.

Bacteria has an interesting role in both our wellness and our illness. They are essential to our existence and make up the majority of our microflora in the digestive tract, yet if the wrong bacteria are allowed to grow in large numbers, they also can cause significant illness. Common bacterial illnesses are associated with ear infections, bladder infections, strep throat, food poisoning and pneumonia. Bacteria can also cause several chronic issues like: SIBO (small intestine bacterial overgrowth), acne, reoccurring acute infections (ear, throat, bladder, etc.), stomach Helicobacter pylori infections or Lyme disease.

There is much research going on today focusing on understanding how these tiny single cell organisms affect our bodies in such an intricate manner. There are literally thousands of bacterial strains in the digestive tract, and any change in their balance has a huge impact on our overall health. Scientists are increasingly linking the alteration of bacterial makeup of the gut with diseases like diabetes, cancer, autism and heart disease. It has even been claimed that our digestive tracts are like our second brain, with the flora acting as the signals. So obviously we have a very tightly linked destiny with these little guys.

In fact, did you know that the origins of our mitochondria (the little energy factories in all of our cells) are bacterial? There is actually separate bacterial DNA present in the mitochondria that regulates its function. Incredible. We do need these guys! So clearly, just taking endless amounts of antibiotics or using anti-bacterial soaps to fight off the "bad" bacteria really isn't doing us any favours long term. Although in the short term, a well-timed antibiotic can save a life, long term and repetitive use of antibiotics sets our system up for disaster.

But wait, didn't I just say I treat chronic bacterial infections? Yes, but a pharmaceutical antibiotic would be a last resort, because the resultant damage to all the flora would undoubtedly make the state of the body worse. My first line defense in a chronic bacterial infection is rarely an antibiotic. For example, I commonly treat Lyme-associated bacterial infections with great success using powerful herbs, like Artemisia or Cat's Claw, that are much more synergistic with gut flora than antibiotics. These remedies are effective at killing off the infection without harming the rest of the body.

Quite often when I see chronic bacterial infections, it is a constant reactivation of the same infection. An example would be a bacterial infection that is plaguing your child's ear over and over again and is never really being cleared. This is also commonly the case with recurrent bladder infection – the body is never fully eradicating the original bacteria.

Often an antibiotic will treat the acute infectious state, but the bacteria is then thrust into a dormant state or biofilm due to the threat of being attacked by the antibiotic, where it readies and waits for the next outbreak opportunity. So, when a chronic bacterial infection is present, it is always important to treat biofilm as well (as discussed earlier in this chapter). I'll use an appropriate form of enzymes to break up the matrix of the biofilm, then allow the immune system and/or antimicrobial treatment to do its work. I see this scenario so often in children with reoccurring bronchitis or strep throat – it is chronic and repetitive because of the biofilm.

Bacteria is also an organism that can make morphology changes (polymorphism). It can change its shape and cellular structure so that it becomes unrecognizable by the immune system. For example, in Lyme disease the Borrelia bacteria changes into a cyst form, and the body's antimicrobial attack then becomes ineffective. In this circumstance, many different types of antibacterial agents will need to be used, that can target the different forms. As previously stated, Grapefruit seed extract, Berberine, or Metronidazole are common cyst busters.

With Susie, we proceeded on a two year course of rotating some antibiotics, herbs, immune support, and biofilm treatment – all the while managing her symptoms with complementary treatment. Particularly with Lyme patients, you have to discern when symptoms surface again whether (1) the treatment is no longer effective, (2) there is another infection you are dealing with, or (3) they're not able to handle the treatment. It's a constant juggling act, and patients that go through treatments with chronic bacterial infections are definitely courageous human beings.

Treatment of these chronic bacterial infections can be so difficult – there is a necessity to keep the good probiotic bacteria flourishing, while at the same time trying to kill the pathogenic bad guys. Not an easy task. Fortunately, as time goes on, the symptoms and treatments get easier. Susie's treatment followed a typical pathway. My first goal in Lyme is to control infection. We then strengthen and build the immune system, often through dealing with other root causes like heavy metals, toxins and nutrient deficiencies. Next, when the patient is strong enough, we start to encourage that infection to become active by breaking up the biofilm, so that we will finally get the upper hand on removing the pathogenic Lyme bacteria.

When we finally got to the point where Susie's infection was testing clear, we did a happy dance! We then began the ongoing work of stabilizing her immune system through the process of immune modulation and healing the resultant damage to systems and flora.

The bottom line is that bacteria are an essential part of our existence. We are required to keep it in a healthy balance. A C. difficile infection after antibiotic use is a perfect example of what can happen when we upset that balance. C. difficile is a normal common bacterium in everyone's digestive tract. However, it is largely unaffected by many antibiotics. So when we take an antibiotic and wipe out a large percentage of the bacterial flora, we make room for the resistant C. difficile to overpopulate. In this circumstance, we don't actually get *exposed* to a bacterium, we literally *remove* some healthy flora, allowing C. difficile to grow and cause an infection. Anyone who has had C. difficile knows this infection is not pleasant, with explosive diarrhea and severe abdominal pain being par for the course. It is often conventionally very difficult to treat. Probiotics are proving to be the most effective treatment, including the most interesting and potent probiotic... fecal transplants!

Might other infections also be caused by an imbalance? Often, whether or not we get an infection is due to too many bacteria in the wrong place or at the wrong time. Is there a potential for a bacterium to get into the *wrong place,* where our immune system won't be prepared for it, leading to an infection? This could occur with something like surgery or dental work. Or if I'm already run down, perhaps from fighting a previous virus or dealing with acute stress, is this the *wrong time* to be exposed to bacteria that could lead to infection? If we use this new formula – bacteria plus wrong place or wrong time equals infection – we can better judge our susceptibility. These would be situations where sterilization and cleanliness would be imperative to prevent bacterial overgrowth. We can choose to do this at times when we are susceptible, rather than constantly using a form of sterilization, like antibacterial soaps, when our risks are quite low.

Common symptoms of bacterial infections:

1. Fevers	2. Yellow sputum
3. Redness, heat and swelling in joints or skin	4. Inflammation
5. Fatigue	6. Diarrhea
7. Repetitive acute infections	8. Chronically enlarged lymph nodes
9. Night sweats	10. Joint and/or muscle pain
11. Headaches	12. Brain fog, poor memory, cognitive symptoms

There is often an emotional message when we experience a bacterial infection. In general, you may feel fixated and experience difficulties with change. You may also feel that you crave attention from others, and feel oversensitive, insecure or vulnerable. Inna Segal of *"The Secret Language of Your Body"* reports people may feel weak, threatened and easily influenced – though they can equally feel frustrated, critical and irritated. Keep in mind, this can occur both ways, the *infection* can lead to these feelings, or these *feelings* can lead to an infection.[6] Dr. Lipton writes and lectures about the significance of how we feel about things being just as (if not more) important than the physical environment our cells are exposed to, including infections.[46] How can that be? The distinction lies in the roots of the disease – are they more emotional or more physical? As we shift into Part 2 later on in this book, you will come to understand that the symptoms you are experiencing will only improve when you've reached the right level of healing. For some people an antibacterial agent is enough – for others, we have to go deeper – perhaps into shifting perspectives, stress management, clearing emotional blocks or changing belief systems.

Susie, like many Lyme patients, discovered an awareness of herself through her healing journey. She worked through past hurts by healing family dynamics and developing a framework of forgiveness. She also found a real sense of purpose. It may be hard to understand, but many of my patients with Lyme disease, once coming through their healing, refer to their experience as a gift. The wisdom they gained from their journey gave them so much more than simply destroying the infection –they courageously overcame their obstacles and found their cure! Susie's experience led her to go on to train as a Holistic Nutritionist so she could help others with Lyme disease and be inspired by her courageous health journey. She has since spoken all over North America and has encouraged many others to look for the answers to their health obstacles. It was a real honour to work with Susie. She was and continues to be so motivated to heal all levels of herself, and even get in touch with her spiritual purpose!

Virus:

When thirty-nine-year-old Bridget came into my office she had been through several medical doctors with no clear answers to what was ailing her, but she was determined to keep looking. She had no diagnosis and was only given bioidentical hormone replacement therapy (BHRT) to help her symptoms of irregular periods. In fact, she had been referred to me by an open-minded MD who felt that BHRT would not solve her significantly low white blood cell count, and she needed a different perspective on healing. Hence she found herself sitting across from me (where people often end up when they've exhausted all other means, unfortunately). Although she couldn't pinpoint for sure when her symptoms started, she felt that within the previous six months she had developed much more severe, debilitating fatigue. Her exhaustion was so significant that she was needing constant naps. She had mild headaches, numbness in her arms and legs that seemingly appeared at random, as well as shortness of breath, sore throat and pressure in her chest. She also suffered from brain fog, dizziness, confusion and forgetfulness. These symptoms were significantly affecting her ability to work and live.

She had done some homework and was pretty sure she had Lyme disease. I certainly didn't rule it out when we first began our investigations, but after going through her history, it didn't seem to fit. She had always been relatively healthy, but her stress levels had been significantly higher in the past few years with marital stress, teenage drama, a move and even a career change. She admittedly had been burning the candle at both ends. When we began discussing when the symptoms had started, she revealed she had had a significant "cold" prior, but that this didn't surprise her too much since she had been so run down. However, it was shortly after this cold when all these other symptoms began to appear. I was able to determine that she was actually fighting a chronic virus, not bacteria. She had Mono when she was younger, and so had her MD run Cytomegalovirus (CMV) and Epstein Barr (EBV) titer blood tests, both of which can cause Mono acutely. Sure enough, her results indicated reactivation of CMV in her system.

Viruses are the smallest microorganisms I discuss in this book. Some viruses are extremely common, like the common cold or influenza, and some are much rarer – like SARS, Ebola or Polio. Viruses are different than all the other microorganisms we have already discussed because they do not have a cell structure. Rather, they are a protein that invades our cells. They then incorporate themselves into our genetic material and replicate through the normal process of protein synthesis. Therefore, once cells are invaded, more viruses are produced, which then go out and attack other healthy cells. This process continues until our immune system is able to stop the virus in its tracks.

Some viruses mutate quickly and tend to cause many rounds of the same illness. Ever wonder why you get the flu more than once in a year? You won't get sick from the same flu virus – rather, it has mutated into a form that is altered enough that your body can't recognize it, so you may get sick a second time. Some viruses mutate very slowly, however, and can linger around in the system for a long time. An example of this is the HIV virus. It mutates once it is attached to an immune cell and eventually evolves into the patient developing AIDS. Herpes viruses, like cold sores or shingles, also evolve by hanging out on nerves and waiting until we're run down enough to start propagating again. This is often why people assume that when they are infected by viruses like genital herpes, they cannot be cleared permanently. Luckily, many medications and supplements are available to slow this replication and prevent outbreak.

With Bridget, we started on immune builders, adrenal support and antiviral treatment. She started to see a change in her energy almost right away. We then added in hydrogen peroxide IVs weekly, which is a super-charged therapy for viruses. We also paired cAMP injections (adenosine monophosphate) alongside this to push the virus out and make the hydrogen peroxide

IVs more effective. With every IV her strength and energy improved, and all of the cognitive symptoms began to dissipate. It was remarkable how quickly she shifted. After two months we were able to discontinue the IV treatments, and her energy and health continued to improve. Whether she went on to make further changes in her life and continue the path of healing, I am not sure, as she stopped coming in (which is often the case with patients once symptoms have resolved). But I always encourage my patients to push beyond the symptoms. Just because the symptoms stop, it doesn't mean we've achieved optimal wellness – which should always be our goal. Moving towards the good things we want – vitality, energy, abundance – not just avoiding the things we don't want – pain, discomfort, fear.

Viruses particularly love the nervous system, and they are often found on nerves. This is something I had to work on in my own healing while recovering from lesions on my brain (diagnosed as MS). After I had Mono, strep throat and tonsillitis at age sixteen (which landed me in the hospital right after New Year's... ick) I can distinctly say that my energy levels and immune system were never the same. I became run down more easily and started to experience dizziness periodically in my twenties without a clear understanding why. I also had massively enlarged tonsils and was prone to frequent throat infections. I saw my MD, a neurologist, and a cardiologist; none of which gave me any answers for the dizziness. I started reading books and magazines on health, and shifted my focus in university to health, fitness and psychology. I started managing the dizziness by eating a more balanced diet of protein, carbs and fats, and avoided all forms of stimulants and caffeine. The experience of dealing with these health mysteries played a part in the choice of my profession as a Naturopathic Doctor. Although these symptoms were very challenging, it wasn't until this virus became active enough, some thirteen years after my initial infection, that the neurological damage was produced by the "perfect storm" of a lingering infection, food intolerances, environmental toxicity and acute trauma. I was merely managing, not clearing the infection, hence I retained the virus as one of the root causes to the more severe neurological disease. Within the healing process, I had to use numerous deeper viral treatments, including healing my tonsils, to help myself finally begin to shift the virus in the right direction.

Common symptoms of viruses:

1. Persistent fevers	2. Clear to opaque sputum
3. Numbness and tingling	4. Dizziness and light headedness
5. Chronic fatigue	6. Fibromyalgia
7. Skin vesicles, hives	8. Recurrent infections
9. Low lymphocyte count	

Emotionally, with viruses we may feel out of control, vulnerable and attacked. We may feel like a victim to circumstance and unable to see our way out. Life may feel chaotic. We may inadvertently seek to control to find balance because of those internal feelings. Again, I use this emotional reference as both a cause and/or effect. The more we work to shift our perspectives to find peace, balance and positivity, the less we will be afflicted or affected by viruses and other ailments.[47] You may not always be able to control an infection, but you can control your outlook on life.

Summary

I hope that through reading this chapter, you now have a better understanding not only of what infectious microbes are, but how our immune system deals with them. Important points are:

1. We need to understand the distinct difference between an acute and chronic infection. Both are relevant to our health but should be treated differently.
2. We need to recognize that infections can become chronic when (1) our immune system is imbalanced, (2) we have persistent exposure, (3) we are dealing with infected root canals, (4) they are harboured in biofilm or (5) they change their morphology.
3. Infections can be distinguished by the microorganism causing

the imbalance: Parasite, Fungus, Bacteria and Virus.

4. Infections can certainly plague us with various symptoms, and it would be easy to label the microorganism as the bad guy. But I want to challenge you to think of these organisms as messengers – here to help you understand your story. They too were created with a distinct purpose. Only when we shift the way we think about these bugs will we really start to understand them.

So, while acknowledging the need for treating and clearing infections, it important that we always ask ourselves, why is the infection there in the first place? What is its purpose? And what can you change physically, emotionally or mentally to bring yourself back into balance?

I want to remove the fear around infections, because our immune system is way more resilient, evolved and intelligent than any microbe it comes in contact with. Have faith in the inherent nature of your body to handle microorganisms. We must learn to both respect their nature and also thrive alongside these little messengers. We cannot nor should not look to just eradicate them all, without examining their deeper purpose. Our immune system holds the key to enable us to deal with these bugs and will ultimately help us understand our complete health journey.

FIVE

Electromagnetic Frequencies

"There are many examples of the failure to use the precautionary
principle in the past, which have resulted in serious and often
irreversible damage to health and environments. Appropriate,
precautionary and proportionate actions taken now to avoid plausible
and potentially serious threats to health from EMF are likely to be
seen as prudent and wise from future perspectives."
~ *European Environment Agency[48]*

The topic of electromagnetic frequencies is confusing for many
people. We are becoming more and more reliant on wireless technology, but at what cost? Is there a cost on our health? We certainly don't
want to end up in a situation where, decades later, we see the failure
of current policies around EMFs, as we did with the harms from
denying the health hazards of smoking, or suggesting pesticides like
DDT or agent orange were safe.

Few governments and organizations seem to take a definitive stance
on the safety of radiation to public health from electromagnetic
devices; however, some science and clinical evidence appears to
suggest concerns. Although there is much debate, the controversial

BioInitiatives Report of 2012 analyzed the research and was able to make correlations: "Bioeffects are clearly established and occur at very low levels of exposure to electromagnetic fields and radiofrequency radiation... Bioeffects can also occur from just minutes of exposure to mobile phone masts (cell towers), WI-FI, and wireless utility 'smart' meters that produce whole-body exposure." The report also states that "Many of these bioeffects can reasonably be presumed to result in adverse health effects if the exposures are prolonged or chronic. This is because they interfere with normal body processes (disrupt homeostasis), prevent the body from healing damaged DNA, produce immune system imbalances, metabolic disruption and lower resilience to disease across multiple pathways."[49]

Tammy came to my office complaining of insomnia and mild depression that seemed to start out of nowhere. She had noticed some menopausal hormone changes, increased stress and slight weight gain, but they seemed to be gradual. In our conversation, we discovered that her Wi-Fi modem was in her bedroom, and she often left her computer and phone on beside her bed. She had moved a few months ago and had set up her house rather quickly, but never really thought of the technology placement as causing a problem. So, I loaned her an EMF reader to go home and look for the signals in her bedroom. She was stunned – the readings were off the chart.

The realization that EMFs have negative health consequences may be overwhelming, so let's examine them more closely. We will look further into their possible effects, but let's first get really clear about what electromagnetic frequencies are and why they are a concern.

WHAT ARE EMFs?

Electromagnetic frequencies (or EMFs) are not a new invention that was created in the technological age. In fact, there are several natural EMFs that are very helpful in governing our environment that we all witness each and every day. From electrical fields that are felt in a lightning storm, to the static cling that we feel in our clothes, to the ability to navigate north versus south by the earth's magnetic pull – all these phenomena occur due to EMFs. Similarly, pilots and frequent fliers may also have increased radiation risks because of their consistent closer proximity to the sun (the major emitter of UV radiation). The entire colour spectrum is actually a part of the natural EMF fields! But outside of colour, we cannot see EMFs around us. Imagine what it would look like to see all the waves from every cell phone, WiFi tower or radio wave around you! That's likely all we would see!

There is a huge spectrum of electric and magnetic fields around us, with some being more damaging than others. The colour spectrum (visible light) is actually what separates frequencies from more damaging to less damaging (see diagram below).

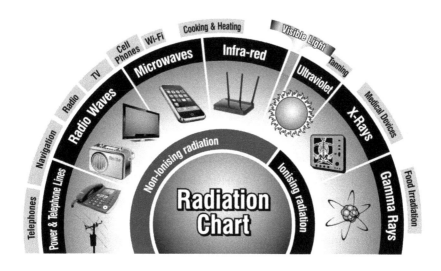

There are also many man-made frequencies that have been added to our environmental mix. Higher frequency radiation, such as the type used in an X-ray machine, has the ability to break cellular bonds and cause damage in our bodies. This is why it is important for us to limit our exposure to X-rays, CT scans and mammograms, as they do pose risks to our cells when overused. Items using lower frequencies include radios, microwaves, ultrasounds, cell phone towers and electrical power lines. For a long time, these waves were believed to pose very little risk to our health – and when our exposure to these frequencies is limited, this is very likely the case. However, with advances in the technological age our exposures have become exponential. We are now almost constantly exposed to low frequency electromagnetic radiation (EMR), and this fact has generated much concern about what the potential health hazards may be.

Since the electrical energy we're talking about is the relationship between atoms and electrons, the fundamental elements which make up all matter, then it's also important to understand that we too, along with all plants and animals, also have resonating frequencies. All living things emit low-level light, heat and acoustical energy, forming electrical and magnetic fields (otherwise known as a biofield). However, how to measure our human biofield is largely disputed, with no real consistency.

"At our most elemental, we are not a chemical reaction, but an energetic charge. Human beings and all living things are a coalescence of energy in a field of energy connected to every other thing in the world. This pulsating energy field is the central engine of our being and our consciousness, the alpha and the omega of our existence."[50]

The human body is incredibly complex, and it depends on the intricately linked electrical and magnetic fields for the functions of life. These fields are associated with heart function, blood and lymph flow and nerve impulses in the brain. They signal molecular transport across cell membranes in order to send messages to cells. There are also many ways that conventional medicine uses the body's electrical frequencies in tests – such as electrocardiograms (ECG) and electroencephalograms (EEG).

Energetic medicines like acupuncture have been treating illnesses for centuries through the maneuvering and manipulation of our biofield. Science is only beginning to understand this energetic principle that has been practiced for so long without a modern method to test its apparent efficacy. Traditional medicines have shown that electrical and magnetic fields are essential, as we can improve health through manipulating our energetic field – therefore, when we are exposed to stronger frequencies, we can also be negatively impacted. We can reason that we are influenced by these higher electromagnetic frequencies because they interact with our own biofield.

HOW DO EMFs AFFECT US?

Tammy went home, moved the WiFi out of her room, and turned off all of her devices in the bedroom. Amazingly, she was able to sleep again! She didn't even realize she had also been suffering from mild headaches until she didn't have them anymore. We still had some concerns around adrenal and digestive health, but how could we ever restore other areas in the body if she was not sleeping? Sleep is a critical parasympathetic function that is needed to repair and heal – a significant requirement to health and wellbeing. She was able to shift her troublesome symptoms almost instantaneously by turning off her electronics. I often see problems with sleeping, frequent colds and flus, headaches, low energy and dizziness as symptoms of EMF exposure. Looking out for and turning off electronic devices can be the turning point for a person's health.

Research regarding EMF exposure has been showing significant trends, according to the BioInitiative Report, who reviewed 325 papers from 2007-2017:

> Several thousand scientific studies over four decades point to serious biological effects and health harm from EMF and RFR (Radio Frequency Radiation). These studies report genotoxicity, single- and double-strand DNA damage... loss of DNA repair capacity in human stem cells, reduction in free-radical scavengers (particularly melatonin), abnormal gene transcription, neurotoxicity, carcinogenicity, damage to sperm morphology and function, effects on behavior, and effects on brain development in the fetus of human mothers that use cell phones during pregnancy... Three meta-analyses have shown significant elevation in rates of childhood leukemia in relation to residential exposure to electromagnetic fields. (BioInitiative Report, 2012)[51]

Evidence has clearly shown that children are more susceptible to radiation than adults. As outlined in The Presidential Cancer Panel, it found "children are at a special risk due to their smaller body mass and rapid physical development, which magnify their vulnerability to known carcinogens, including radiation."[52] Since children are disproportionally affected by EMR, our regulations of allowable limits from most devices are largely unacceptable for children.

This is even more important to understand as our kids grow up in an increasingly technologically connected world. They are exposed to WiFi often both at home and at school, and often frequently use cell phones or smartphones. Clinically, I have seen numerous children who have come into the office with complaints ranging from headaches, to difficulty sleeping, poor concentration, stomachaches and behavior problems. After assessment, I have often suspected high EMF and WiFi exposures, and have the parent use our EMF meter to measure their exposures at home and even at school. Time and time again, the readings come up high. And typically, that is just from WiFi modem, electrical devices or smart meter locations in the home, not the added use of mobile devices. It's remarkable the differences I have seen in children when the EMF devices are removed or shut off. A relatively simple change!

One such example was little four-year-old Ryder. He was experiencing symptoms of poor sleep, hyperactivity and tics. His mom also reported he had a hard time staying focused, and temper tantrums were still a significant issue for him when things didn't go his way. I suspected EMFs when I tested him in the office, so I suggested his mom take home the EMF reader to assess his bedroom. Sure enough, she was surprised that there were high levels in his room, since it wasn't close to the Wi-Fi box or smart meter. They were particularity high over his bed! She started turning things off, to no avail – until she turned off the breaker to his bedroom, then noticed the meter was finally signaling a normal reading. So, each and every night she turned off his breaker. In a few short weeks, his behavior was calmer, he was sleeping through the night and his head tic stopped! It was that quick and easy!

I do believe we are all affected by EMFs, as human beings are all inherently the same – the individual difference being that we are each affected to varying degrees. I have seen clinically that the more imbalanced, or "sick" a person is, the more likely they will notice the effects of electromagnetic radiation on their health. I have patients that find their chronic symptoms such as rampant headaches, reduced immunity, insomnia, chronic pain and decreased cognitive function are aggravated when they are exposed to EMFs.

The BioInitiative Report in both 2007 and 2012 included both human and animal studies that showed evidence of EMFs causing these effects: [53]

• Disruption of homeostasis (normal cellular function)
• Prevention of DNA healing[54]
• Immune system imbalances and lowered resilience to infections
• Headaches[55]
• Sleep disturbances[56]
• Effects on sperm quality, mobility, and repair and infertility [57]
• Induced stress response[58]
• Associated with hyperactivity and autism in children where mothers had high exposure[59]
• Impact on melatonin production,[60]
• Changed enzymes affecting DNA and cell growth[61]
• Associated with increased risk of brain tumors[62]
• Accentuated environmental toxicity (similar to heavy metals)
• Generated free radicals that damage DNA[63]
• Neuro-hormone changes, which can result in memory loss and impaired brain function.[64]

The majority of the population has completely overlooked the vast number of negative effects of EMFs. I felt broaching this topic in my book was essential because EMFs are a contributing root cause of disease. Our society is becoming increasingly more dependent on electronics for basic everyday functions. It is highly unlikely the demand for electrical devices will decrease in our future. So it is our responsibility to be aware and cognizant of how we can mitigate our individual sources of EMFs to the best of our ability. They are an invisible toxic influence that if left unchecked, under-tested and unregulated, could lead us down a path of overexposure that would be very difficult to reverse. Knowledge is power – being able to diminish the influence of EMFs in the lives of you and your family gives you some control over this circumstance.

A Note on Geopathic Stress

Geopathic stresses are earth magnetic frequencies that are created underground from the flow of ground water. When one area of ground water flows across another, it creates a magnetic field. These areas are a normal occurrence and are everywhere around us. They are areas where ant hills form, cats gravitate to and trees grow away from. For the most part they are not an issue for our health, unless we are spending a lot of time directly over them – most commonly, in an area that you are sleeping in or working in day after day.

There is evidence from Europe that shows that where people stay in the same home for decades, often sleeping in the same place in the home, that they were more prone to disease development in the areas of the body that were directly over a geopathic stress zone. Hence, mapping out your bedroom for stress zones can be significant. Often you simply need to change the wall the bed is on, or even just move it over a few inches. Geopathic stress zones are quite small, but they are also numerous. They can easily be found by using curved metal rods in the same way a water well is found, because it's the same principle! Holding the rods parallel and watching for them to cross, or magnetically attract to each other, is how geopathic stresses are found. Much like EMFs then, when chronic, they can affect our health. We are energetic, so anything that affects our internal frequencies can be detrimental.

Summary

1. Electromagnetic frequencies are unseen forces of influence on humans and our environment.
2. Some EMFs can be helpful – like heat, sound and light – but they can also be harmful – like microwaves, UV rays and X-rays.
3. With continuous increases in technology, we are seeing correlated increases in EMF exposures.
4. We are all being affected by these frequencies – to what degree depends on our usage, age and health status.
5. Mitigating our exposures is key – by turning technology off, using wired-in options or using grounding devices. We will go into more details about these options in Part 2 of the book.

SIX

Stress and Trauma

"Stress is not what happens to us. It's our response to what happens.
And *response* is something we can choose."
~ *Maureen Killoran*

For many people, stress is encountered on a regular basis and doesn't require an explanation. However, I'd like to fully define what stress actually is before we move on to how it affects us. By definition, stress is "the non-specific response of the body to any demand placed upon it," according to Dr. Hans Selye.[65] We can expand on this description with the explanation that basically every time our body has to adapt to its environment, it sets off a chain reaction to respond to that demand. This stressor could be anything – running from a cougar, fighting an infection, driving in traffic or even just standing up from a chair – the body has to adapt all its bodily functions to that perceived threat or requirement.

All animals (well, at least mammals) have the capacity for stress, an automatic triggered response. This response allows them to "fight or flight" in order to survive. It ultimately perceives some sort of threat, and in order to survive, it must respond. This means 100% of the body's focus shifts to the stress response, completely shutting down relaxation and healing. And although too much stress for prolonged periods of time can be detrimental, we must also remember it is necessary. We require a certain amount of stress to adjust to our environment. It is both adaptive and healthy. We are meant to have a balance between stress and relaxation, with no more than 50% of our body functioning in sympathetic stress response the majority of the time, so that we can reach homeostasis or balance.

The difference between humans and other animals, according to the book *Why Zebras Don't Get Ulcers*, is that humans have the ability to anticipate stress even if we're not in a stressful situation.[66] How does this affect us? We can just *think* about a situation that we deem stressful, like an argument we had with our spouse or the fear of an upcoming deadline, and get the same physiological response as if a cougar was actually chasing us!

So as much as the unique cognitive capacity of our intellectual minds is a gift, we are also cursed with need to be *mindful* of what's going on up there. We can trigger a stress reaction in our body not only by a physical event but also by a mental one! This is a big reason why people are living in more of an 80:20 or 90:10 stress to relaxation balance – not because they're actually in a stressful event but rather they're thinking of one. And the statistics associated with this high level of stress and disease are staggering. According to the Center for Disease Control and Prevention for the United States, it has been estimated that 75% of all visits to primary care physicians are for stress related problems: fatigue, digestive concerns, pain, headaches, mood disorders or anxiety, for example. Occupation Health and Safety puts that number up to 90%.[67] Therefore, the goal of stress management should always be looking to achieve that balance. The circadian rhythm is defined as a cycle of balance – where we wake up in the morning and feel refreshed and ready for the day (when the stress hormone cortisol is higher), but then at night we feel more relaxed and finally ready for a good night's sleep to heal and rejuvenate (when cortisol is lower).

The Physiology of Stress:

So what is stress actually doing to our bodies that it has such a huge impact? When our body is exposed to a stressful circumstance, it triggers two responses – the first from the autonomic nervous system, the second from the hormonal system. The immediate response to a stress trigger comes from the former, the autonomic nervous system. This system is divided into two separate pathways – one that triggers a stress response, the sympathetic nervous system, and the second that triggers relaxation, the parasympathetic nervous system. The second response (the latter of the two responses - the hormonal system) is the "backup" so to speak, to the immediate autonomic nerve response. The systems and their pathways respond in the following order:

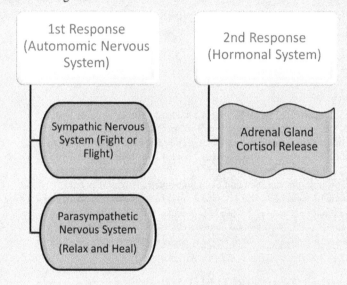

1. Sympathetic Nervous System

This pathway of the autonomic system is much faster than the responses from the hormonal system, as the first responder to stress. Imagine we're in Pamplona, Spain, and a herd of incensed bulls are running towards us! The sympathetic nervous system is triggered! It consists of a compilation of successive nerves along the spine, and releases a neurotransmitter called acetylcholine. These nerves from the spine all end up at different target organs or tissue, and subsequently release the neurotransmitters epinephrine and norepinephrine, initiating the primitive fight or flight response. As the bulls approach we start sweating, our heart rate goes up, our blood pressure increases, our pupils dilate, our lung bronchi open up, our muscles are fueled with blood, our vessels constrict to move the blood where we need it, and we stop digesting our delicious Seafood Paella lunch to shunt the blood to more important areas. This adrenaline rush is familiar to most people, such as in the example of a person having superhuman strength to lift up a car to save someone who is trapped. Or in this example, to run like crazy in front of an angry, snorting herd of bulls!

2. Hormonal System

The second reaction in a stress response is the hormonal response, where the adrenal gland secretes cortisol. The pituitary gland in the brain stimulates the adrenal cortex to produce cortisol in times of perceived stress. Since hormones are transported in the blood, they tend to have a slightly slower onset, but their effects can last longer. Cortisol effects the body by releasing blood sugar from our liver stores so that we have sustained energy to react. This allows us to continue running from the bull past the point of our adrenaline wearing off in order to get into a place of safety.

The physiological response to stress occurs in every human as an essential process in life. However, the typical person now experiences a stressful event an average of thirty-five times in a day! Wow, no wonder we are seeing problems.

3. Parasympathetic Nervous System

The "non-stress functions," those that are not part of immediate survival of self, are controlled by the parasympathetic nervous system, and other hormones like DHEA. They are only activated when we are *not* in stress. These functions include digestion, sleep, healing, immune function, metabolism and reproduction – which are all inhibited by the presence of stress. They are inherently important for survival in the long term. If we were always running from that bull, or maybe other perceived bullies, we would constantly be shutting down our digestion, metabolism, immune function and even hormone balance. A lack of parasympathetic functions would threaten the existence of our whole human race! Often when patients are experiencing problems such as hormone imbalances, repetitive infections, poor wound healing, unexplained weight gain, insomnia or digestive complaints, it is safe to say that stress is playing a role.

HYPERADRENISM: "TIRED BUT WIRED"

When Travis, aged 35, came into my office he was a wreck. He wasn't sleeping, and he seemed to have little patience for anything. His biggest complaint, however, was the fact that his muscle and sexual stamina was dramatically diminished. He was going through a major change in his life with starting up a new company in the last couple years and was managing several people in that process. He was juggling the start of this new business, his finances, and taking care of his kids as a part time single parent. He was losing passion for this new found venture and couldn't stop his mind from overanalyzing every situation. He used to find an outlet in exercise but recently, it seemed to make him worse. His medical doctor noticed his blood pressure seemed to be rising and had told him blood pressure medications may be in his near future if things didn't change. When I asked him if he was stressed, he actually said not any more than usual, but he had gone through a separation recently that left him drained.

I see overstressed individuals in my office on a weekly, if not daily, basis. Overstimulation, or *hyperadrenism*, where the cortisol levels become too high, is a typical response to too much stress. The body is over-responding. The person feels like they are chronically in a state of stress, and for all intents and purposes, they are.

I often use the analogy of a water tank to describe the capacity of your body to handle stress. Imagine that every day you fill that water tank with the water supply that you need to survive, and as long as you fill the same or more than you take, you will never run out. Imagine that you fill that water tank as full as you will need each day – based on the quality of your diet, sleep, nutrients and vitamins – and then you drain from it when you need the energy supply to react to a situation.

Now picture that your water demand goes way up, say if you are working harder or it's hotter outside, and you open that tap full blast. You are taking more water each time than you allotted for when you filled the tank. What's more, sometimes you forget to turn the tap off after you have finished drinking. Your body still perceives an inevitable threat and thus the adrenal tank thinks you're still in high demand mode. It gets stuck on.

This is very common. Not only do we have this excess cortisol in our system when we're in the stressful situation, but in an overstressed individual, it can also remain after the acute stress is over. Examples where this may occur include grief or divorce – the body perceives the stressor is still there because our minds are consciously or unconsciously recalling the stressful event.

After interviewing my new patient Travis and hearing about all the stressors he was currently experiencing, I instinctively felt that cortisol was the first culprit we would have to address. I tested him in my office using salivary hormone testing, as blood tests are not the best way to assess cortisol. (If you don't have a biofeedback testing method, salivary or urinary hormone testing is best.) His cortisol was extremely high. We started a supplement called phosphatidylserine, a natural phospholipid found in the body that assists in sending the message to the adrenal gland that "there is no stress now." The typical dose of 200-400 mg was successful to decrease his cortisol levels and get his system regulated again. He noticed in a couple of nights that not only was he sleeping better, and through the night, but he seemed a lot calmer and more capable to problem solve. Eventually his blood pressure started to shift in a positive direction, and his energy and stamina started to improve. Of course, in order to maintain these improvements, a shift in his perspective or situation would be essential to permanently reduce the stress, not just treat the symptoms.

The most common symptom that people report in this phase is feeling "tired but wired," where they are constantly feeling drained, but there is no way their body will let them relax. They feel like they're treading water and barely staying afloat, where any small stressful event can be completely overwhelming, making them feel like they might drown. They have trouble shutting off their brain; they feel anxious. Sleep is a futile task. They may have little appetite, and/or find they are losing weight, both muscle and fat, without changing anything. It is very important to recognize when this pattern is occurring because the body becomes so concerned about survival that any other health task is completely ignored or ineffective, putting the patient's health at risk.

In playing cards, a wild card or trump suit can win automatically over other cards. Think of cortisol as that dominant card. It overrules all other "suits" or body functions, because it believes if it doesn't respond to the stressor with 100% commitment, you will literally die. The fight or flight response is designed to protect you from harm. It can't tell the difference between a cougar chasing you or forgetting your Aunt Tessie's birthday party. Remember, real or imagined, the body behaves the same way... stress is stress.

Therefore, if we are not cognizant of our chronic stressors, there is the risk that the tank will empty to such a degree that we can no longer get from it what we need, and end up in an adrenal crash or overwhelming fatigue. Before we discuss the specifics of how this process works, understand that the body cannot heal unless it is in a relaxed or opposing parasympathetic state. See the table below for how the pattern of salivary cortisol changes in different scenarios if stress is not addressed.

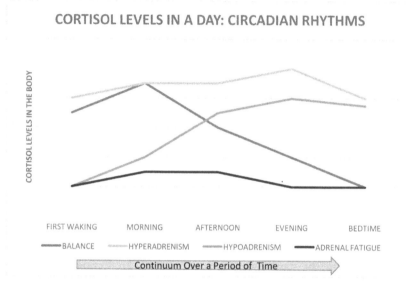

HYPOADRENISM: "TIRED AND EXHAUSTED"

Lacy, aged thirty-four, came into my office struggling. She was a single mother and had recently moved to town. She had little family support here but had decided she needed a new start. The only problem was, she could hardly function. She felt like she was always needing to push herself, and whenever she sat down she would totally crash. She was exhausted, and no amount of sleep seemed to help her. She also had no physical endurance, feeling wiped out for days after exercising. This was especially troubling for her as she used to train intensively for fitness competitions. Her previous workouts were grueling, but now she could hardly go for a simple hike without it causing her whole body to ache. She noticed her periods were becoming more irregular, and her flow seemed heavier. She was also getting more PMS symptoms, which was unusual for her. The changes in menstruation indicated a likely diagnosis of estrogen dominance. Finally, her digestion seemed to be more challenging with daily bloating and gas, and irregular bowels, from constipation to loose stools. It was evident that she had irritable bowel syndrome; however, when looking at the overall picture, it was clear that the root of the problems was chronic stress, and the resultant under-functioning adrenals. She was quite literally pushing herself into further exhaustion trying to keep up.

So what happens when the stress becomes chronic, ongoing and constant? Your body will do its best to compensate and adjust, but at some point the body's resilience and reserves become depleted. People who have reached this point describe feeling exhausted all the time, like they just want to sleep. However, no amount of sleep changes their energy level – while normally sleep could restore them. They are now depleted beyond what a good night's sleep can provide.

Remember that water reservoir? Well, in this situation, the tank is drained so low that you can only get a slow drip out of the tap. If you attempt to stimulate yourself, maybe through being busy, physical activity or caffeine, you might squeeze out a couple more drops, but this will leave the tank even more depleted. In hypoadrenism, or under-responding of the adrenal glands, our body's ability to adapt to stress is low. We are literally not making sufficient amounts of cortisol to produce a normal circadian rhythm (depicted on the chart above as the "balance" rhythm). A normal circadian rhythm has higher cortisol in the morning, so we wake refreshed and ready to go, and lower cortisol at night, so we feel relaxed and ready for a rejuvenating sleep. Again, this is not something you will likely see on a blood test, but a four-point salivary cortisol test would diagnose hypoadrenism more effectively.

The curve on our graph that represents cortisol levels in hypoadrenism goes in the opposite direction to the balanced graph. We wake up exhausted and unrefreshed, then push all day long to gain some energy from external stimuli, due to a lack of an internal source. We then often find we will get a "second wind" or feel overstimulated at night, and have trouble sleeping. This reduction in quality of sleep then further disrupts our healing and rejuvenation processes at night.

Adrenal fatigue has gained more understanding over the past few years, and I would say it is part of the continuum of the development of hypoadrenism – the most severe end of this spectrum. Adrenal fatigue occurs when the body has reached burnout stage, and is now not-responding. The symptoms are often more severe, debilitating and chronic. These cases take much more time and support in order to dig the patient out of the cortisol flatline, as they have no real peaks of energy. This is often when chronic fatigue or fibromyalgia are diagnosed. The good news is that these are both treatable and curable, providing the root cause of the chronic stress is addressed.

There are six key areas in the body affected by the overproduction of cortisol in chronic stress:

1) Digestion

Cortisol influences our digestive capacity. When we are stressed, cortisol is released, adapting our digestion to inhibit the stomach parietal cells to stop the flow of juices or acid. This happens because the body does not want to waste energy digesting a meal if it is about to become one (as in our example of a cougar chasing you)! However, when excess cortisol has been produced over and over again, for months and even years, the body is constantly suppressing stomach acid. The result? A breakdown in the digestive tract.

Stomach acid has several functions in the digestive process:

- it kills pathogens, needed because food is not sterile
- it stimulates motility of the stomach
- it triggers the cardiac sphincter (muscle at the top the stomach) to contract and stay closed so food is not regurgitated

- it initiates the release of mucin, our natural "Pepto Bismol" that coats the stomach lining so we don't begin to digest our organs
- it activates our digestive enzymes in the duodenum of the small intestine to break down further.

As stomach acid has such a large role to play in digestion, when its functions are inhibited, it can cause

- GERD or reflux,
- heartburn (acid in the esophagus, where it should never reach),
- stomach irritation or gastritis,
- heaviness,
- fullness,
- indigestion,
- belching,
- malabsorption,
- nutrient deficiencies,
- infections,
- bloating and
- food sensitivities from a leaky, irritated small intestine.

That covers a lot of digestive symptoms from one root issue, doesn't it?

2) Hormones

The adrenals influence ovaries and testes by supporting or suppressing their function. The presence of cortisol triggers the production of more estrogen in fat cells from the hormones testosterone (influencing stamina and libido) and DHEA (influencing muscle building, repair and anti-aging) in both men and women. Also, since estrogen is a growth hormone, it likes to make us soft and squishy by increasing our fat tissue! Cortisol depletion also reduces progesterone, as it has a similar molecular structure to cortisol.

Because of this, the body can steal progesterone to make cortisol any time the stress demand requires... which furthers the development of estrogen dominance.

Effects of estrogen dominance include

- moodiness,
- breast tenderness,
- irritability,
- weight gain,
- anxiety,
- depression,
- increase in thyroid binding globulin (TBG) to inactive thyroid hormones,
- insomnia,
- change in menses,
- fibroids,
- endometriosis,
- ovarian cysts and
- abnormal tissue growth in breast, uterus or prostate.

3) Thyroid

There are two ways cortisol interferes with thyroid function:

1. The previously discussed estrogen dominance causes a suppression of TSH (thyroid stimulating hormone) which then reduces thyroid hormone production, resulting in hypothyroid type symptoms.
2. Cortisol also influences the conversion of T4 to T3. T4, thyroxin, is our inactive thyroid hormone. It must be converted to T3, triiodothyronine, to become active and affect our metabolism (see diagram below). Therefore, this conversion is extremely important. Under chronic stress, the body slows down metabolism because the adrenals cannot keep up to a high demand. This causes a down regulation of

the thyroid, decreasing TSH and blocking T4 from converting into active T3. Instead, cortisol makes another inactive thyroid hormone called reverse T3 (rT3). This can also be tested in the blood and can be a good marker for cortisol effects on the thyroid.

The reduction in T3 and presence of rT3 can indicate hypothyroidism. The hard part here is that TSH is the only test typically performed conventionally in the blood, which may or may not be correlated to the T3! Hence many patients may go undiagnosed with a normal TSH! This is why to understand this pattern, all thyroid hormones must always be tested to rule out a problem, TSH, T4, and T3. Hypothyroid symptoms include:

- weight gain,
- fatigue,
- depression,
- dry skin,
- cold body temperature and
- constipation.

I believe there are a number of non-autoimmune hypothyroid cases that are actually hypoadrenal cases. The thyroid is just being affected by the adrenals, and then responding perfectly to our intricately connected hormonal system. Hence both systems need to be supported and addressed.

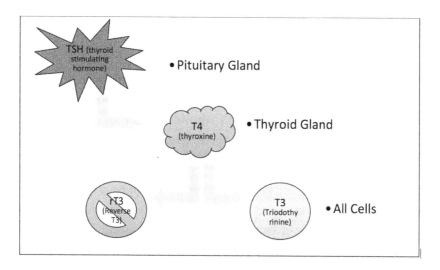

4) Blood sugar

Cortisol is a glucocorticoid, which means it regulates blood sugar. It stimulates the breakdown of fat and muscle to create readily available sugar for the body to fight or take flight. But what happens when we are doing this too often? We start to see blood sugar dysregulation – meaning we are releasing sugar at times that are not related to food intake, and we start to see irregular blood sugar highs and corresponding lows throughout the day. Dysregulated blood sugar can affect your mood and focus, cause headaches and dizziness, and create energy spikes and lows. This is why you can feel "hangry" even when you have been eating regular meals!

What's worse, we are often not burning this energy when we are just thinking about that stressful situation at work, so we store it again, only this time solely as fat! I call it the adrenal inner tube, that extra fat that sits around the waist like a floating device and seems impossible to get rid of, no matter what diet or exercise regime we try.

5) Immune system

Ever wonder why you seem to get sick on holidays and no other time?! Because cortisol alters your immune system! You have probably heard of prednisone, an anti-inflammatory drug, derived to mimic a natural process of high cortisol in the body – but at a much more aggressive level. Cortisone is the natural compound of inactive cortisol! At high levels it naturally suppresses the immune system, or more specifically, inflammation. This is because if you are dealing with immediate survival, healing a wound or fighting an infection is the last thing your body wants to spend energy on. It wants to get you out of immediate danger, then it can work on healing.

Therefore, if the immune system is constantly suppressed, our healing and infection fighting capacity is affected. Remember, the symptoms of a cold or flu are not caused by the bug, but occur because your immune system is working. Just because you don't have symptoms doesn't mean there isn't a bug there you should be clearing, especially when "everyone around you is sick."

Conversely, with chronic stress and low cortisol, the immune system becomes more unregulated, and we may see more inflammation in the body, like arthritis or autoimmune diseases.

Symptoms of immune system dysregulation can include

- allergies,
- frequent infections,
- long standing infections,
- pain,
- never getting "colds or flus,"
- arthritis,
- autoimmune diseases,
- heart disease and
- any type of cancer.

Our bodies are designed to handle roughly 50% stress and 50% relaxation to modulate and balance our immune systems, and when this balance is disrupted, there is no question the immune system will be affected.

6) Sleep

This one probably seems obvious, as most of you know when you're stressed you don't sleep as long and/or your sleep is more disrupted. However, when stress is chronic and you become more tired, it's interesting that your sleep quality is also negatively affected. This happens because cortisol has a direct relationship to melatonin. When cortisol is high, melatonin becomes lower in response. The circadian rhythms of the body require these opposing patterns (see chart above). So, if the stress is chronic, this leads to higher cortisol at night, then the melatonin will naturally be suppressed, not allowing for a rejuvenating sleep.

Disrupted sleep leads to

- fatigue,
- insomnia,
- poor recovery,
- change in moods and
- decreased focus and memory.

As you can see, it is very obvious that sleep cannot be overrated, as it is an essential part of anyone's healing journey. Rest really does equal rejuvenation!

In the case with Lacy, we soon began to turn things around when we started her on some intensive adrenal support, curbed some of her lifestyle habits, and gave her body the space to work on healing. This included needing to cut back on exercise to a more low to moderate intensity and improve her sleep patterns by sleeping at consistent times and in complete darkness. We also worked on balancing her blood sugars as much as possible with a lower glycemic diet. In the end, she didn't go back to intensive training because she realized that it was actually working against her. Instead, she learned to listen to the limits of her body and live a much more balanced life. She could enjoy exercise as long as it didn't start to compromise her energy or recovery.

Athletes have to be particularly mindful of the delicate balance between exercise intensity together with unhealthy stress. Exercise, although extremely beneficial for us, can be a significant stress, especially when training at an elite level. So any additional stresses to those athletes, such as infections, toxins or mental / emotional stress, leave them vulnerable to burnout. They have to be extra diligent to protect their routine of sleep and eating. They need to support healthy adrenal function in order to continue sports at that caliber over the long term.

It is not a coincidence that hands down, the most common symptoms that patients are experiencing when coming into my office are disrupted sleep, energy, digestion and hormones. Each of these is intricately connected to stress. The hard part is, there is no magic pill.

Understand that stress is a universal experience – no one is immune. Over the centuries, the sources of stress have changed to varying degrees, but there really hasn't been a decline in the amount of stress we encounter. However, we also know people have never lived in a time like today, where access to helpful stress-busting resources are everywhere! From relaxation techniques, to self-help books and courses, to life coaches and counsellors, to ample support groups and education – all are there to assist you in changing the stress in your life. We can change our reality. Stress can quickly come, but it can also quickly go (think about the last time you went on a blissful holiday!). The constant striving to make that holiday feeling a permanent reality, whatever your circumstances are, will serve your body more than any magic pill will. In Part 2, I will discuss in detail several strategies for dealing with stress, incorporating many of the levels of healing.

TRAUMA IN RELATIONSHIP TO STRESS

"Every single thing that has ever happened in your life is preparing you for a moment that is yet to come."
~ *Unknown*

First of all, I will start by saying that no one deserves pain, unhappiness and discomfort. Things that happen to people do not happen because at some level they karmically deserved it. We are all human beings – no one's value is different from another, and we all desire love, joy, connection and belonging. It is our birthright. However, sometimes in our path there are struggles that we must defeat. If we don't find a way to deal with a traumatic event, we may breed more troubling events/emotions because of the past energy that we are carrying forward.

By definition, a trauma is an experience or perception of something that is deeply distressing or disturbing to your physical, energetic, emotional or mental bodies. I tend to describe trauma as an intensely stressful event that goes beyond your capacity to cope. This is a very individual experience, so there are no real black and white inclusions or exclusions to what constitutes trauma, but these experiences could include pain, abuse, violence, war, accidents, injuries, severe illness, death, divorce, separation or rejection on any level.

Childhood trauma can be particularly long lasting. Studies by the CDC have even correlated a high number of adverse childhood events to 7 out of the top 10 major causes of disease leading to death![68] Obviously this is significant!

Traumatic events for a child may include

- divorce or separation,
- death of a loved one,
- domestic violence,
- physical, sexual or emotional abuse,
- physical or emotional neglect,
- substance addictions and abuse,
- mental illness in the family,
- bullying,
- physical trauma,
- in utero or birth trauma or stress,

- poverty or homelessness, and
- war or natural disasters

If you become traumatized at a young age, time may inevitably allow you to suppress the experience and even emotionally disassociate from it. We are often not given adequate support or proper resources, nor taught how to deal with these traumas, especially at a young age. Hence the trauma can be internalized, and the body can remember. It ultimately seeps into your current reality, perhaps through feeling fearful, angry or anxious all the time without knowing why. This is how our biography becomes our biology.[69]

Does this mean if you have lived through any of these traumatic experiences, then you are holding onto old trauma? Not necessarily. Sometimes these things actually help shape your perspective and increase your ability to adapt to your surroundings. However, if negative feelings do linger, they may cause unconscious post-traumatic stress. This could, for example, manifest as anxiety; where you are more strongly affected by the fight or flight response in stress. In others it could be connected to other mental health issues.

In cases of abuse, unfortunately often people who inflict the most pain or hurt to others have been the most traumatized in their own lives. These people were children once too, who didn't have the opportunity to overcome their circumstances or find the support to deal with their pain. This can sometimes lead to a viscous cycle of abuse, but absolutely does not have to be the reality.

Post-traumatic stress (PTS) occurs when a traumatic event continues to create stress in the body, sometimes long after the initial event happened. The memory of the incident still has the emotional power to re-traumatize you at any moment, when your brain unconsciously makes a connection to that initial event or situation. This happens because whether the situation is real (actually happening at this time) or imagined (as in a memory), the body responds in the same way. It doesn't know how to tell the difference between past, present or future tense. The physical reacting body is always in the now.

PTS can be especially limiting and debilitating to a person's ability to live and interact in the world free of burden and fears. PTS may bear a whole host of panic, phobia or anxiety disorders.

The key to understanding how to heal trauma is not by looking at *what* we go through but rather *how* we go through it. Essentially, what we do with the memories of the trauma?

We can make all the wise and well-calculated choices in the world, but we can't always avoid "life" happening to us. A traumatic event or situation can deeply impact us and shake us to our core; therefore, naturally it makes sense that trauma is connected to our root causes of illness. To get to the other side of the emotional pain it causes, you have to acknowledge what the trauma is – an energetically charged memory that is robbing you of your power to live in the present moment, healthy and free.

While the event or situation may have been devastating, you can ulti-mately change your perspective –through shifting awareness, coun-selling, forgiveness and many other techniques we will discuss in later chapters. You really can find an opportunity for growth by moving through the emotions connected to the trauma.

The way you perceive or label a situation in your life – as bad, painful or devastating, for example – actually holds you in an internal conflict. These circumstances are a part of your history, but they don't need to define you. When you acknowledge the pain and allow the body to let go of your emotional connection to it through continued work on your healing process, you can redefine your future.

We are not victims; we are conscious creators. We need to find ways to look for and accept the internal growth from what we have experi-enced, working through the hurt, anger, disappointment, fear or betrayal – rather than externalizing the feelings by creating an attitude of blame or judgement of others or ourselves. When we blame others, we take away the opportunity to be responsible for our lives.

This is often coined a victim mentality. This only leaves us feeling jaded or hopeless. We essentially are giving our power over our lives away. If we are resistant to this growth and change in perspective, we limit our ability to fully participate in our own lives and what we create in the future.

Trauma can be a real limitation to a person's ability to heal, but as you will discover in the next few chapters, you can be free from this, no matter how difficult it may seem.

Summary

1. The stress response is an adaptive compensation to something demanding in the body's environment – it could be a physical stress like an injury, structural misalignment, toxicity or infection – or it could also be a mental or emotional stress like an argument, deadline or a fearful event.
2. When the body is in balance, it swiftly responds to the stress, deals with the attack, and then returns to its homeodynamic state of flow and balance.
3. When stress is ongoing, you first move into a chronically high cortisol state, hyperadrenism – but can ultimately end up in a chronically low cortisol state, hypoadrenism, and eventually adrenal fatigue (burnout).
4. Stress physically affects several areas of the body including: digestion, hormones, thyroid support, blood sugar balance, the immune system and sleep.
5. Trauma can be the instigator of chronic stress in our body's system. It is often not fully acknowledged or known by the person affected. Trauma can also lead to dysfunction and disease.
6. Our bodies are designed to support a state of 50% stress and

50% relaxation. We must learn to recognize, support and release the excessive stressors in our lives to be able to achieve an optimal state of wellness.

SUMMARY TO PART I

So, now that we have fully dissected the root causes of disease, we can dive deeper into the levels of healing. As we move forward, it's vitally important to intentionally let go of your past point of view, the one that may make you feel stuck, fearful, helpless and disconnected. Be open to changing your inner dialogue. Every root we have discussed requires actions and changes. This in turn requires that you are willing to wade through the weeds of resistance and break through into a deeper personal understanding.

In other words, when you are open to the challenge of examining your current narrative around your health, you will in turn allow your health journey to evolve. I pray that at this point in the book, you truly understand *why we get sick*, and are ready to receive the tools for your health transformation. To step into *your* courageous cure and know that you can change your story.

Part Two

There Are Levels to Healing: Treatment Must Reach the Right Level

"The greatest medicine of all is teaching people how to not need it."
~Hippocrates

The evolution of medicine and healing was an interesting process in history. From Shaman and medicine men, to folklore, superstitions and spirit possessions, to clergymen and nuns performing medical care – we have seen many variations of healers. We have also had many different cultural and traditional medicines and practices that have stood the test of time and are still being used today, such as herbal medicine or acupuncture. Philosophers and healers like Hippocrates and Galen influenced the understanding of the body and disease for centuries. Few people realize that the current dominant medical model in North America has only been around since the nineteenth century, and pharmaceuticals for roughly 100 years. This current dominant model in North America has been largely developed from a theory that believes your genes are the sole determinant of who you are, and as such, the primary reason for your disease – you are helpless to your disease and there is nothing you can do about it!

It also looks at each part of the body separately rather than a whole, which is why there is a specialist for each area of the body. Hence, we may tend to miss the bigger health picture. Now that you understand the root causes of disease, I am hoping, at this point in the book, that you can see how limiting this approach can be. It is incredibly disempowering. As we have already covered, while your genes are your blueprint, if we base our whole medical model and theory of disease on this fact, many people will unfortunately continue to suffer. This is not to say that there isn't a time or place for conventional medical technologies or innovations, quite the opposite. We have never before been able to save lives in acute situations, like war, natural disasters or accidents, in the way we can now. Through the use of antibiotics, anesthetics, diagnostic testing and even technologically assisted surgeries, lives are saved, limbs repaired and physical trauma healed. However, if we are going to truly heal the body that is suffering from chronic health situations, it is not always about cutting it out, burning it off, or suppressing it. Pharmaceuticals also have a place in treatment, but when they are required long term, understand that they are not fixing the problem – drugs merely manage the symptoms.

In order to heal at a deep level and find your courageous cure, you must ensure that with each root area of imbalance, you seek to heal the body on the appropriate and corresponding level. If we can completely understand the message that the body is trying to convey (it is "speaking" in symptoms, rather than words) then we can eliminate the symptom altogether.

The body has five main levels of healing of which we need to be aware. The descriptions of these levels are based on the theories of many philosophers and ancient cultures throughout history, some of which further subdivide the levels. For simplification and ease of understanding, I explain this basic healing structure as five levels. The framework at which the body heals is as follows:

1. First Level – the physical body: bones, tissues and fluids

2. Second Level – the energetic body: the vital force or Chi that flows through our body
3. Third Level – the emotional body: the perception of our surroundings
4. Fourth Level – the mental body: subconscious and unconscious mind
5. Fifth Level – the spiritual body: connection to God and all living things; light, love and truth

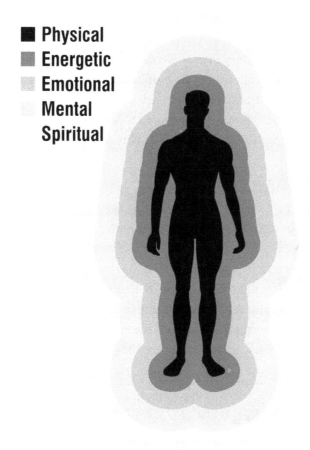

Physical
Energetic
Emotional
Mental
Spiritual

These bodies are present in each and every one of us. They are also hierarchical in nature (see diagram). The most basic and primal level is the physical body, and the most enlightened and impactful is the spiritual essence of the body. The higher up an imbalance occurs the more layers below it that can also be affected. For example if there is an imbalance on the third or fourth level, the more likely the first and second levels will also be impacted. A good way to imagine this is using the analogy of Babushka dolls, borrowed from my good friend Josep Soler, author of *The Art of Listening to Life*.[70] Layers of increasingly larger dolls surround the tiny wooden doll at the center, the physical body. While each bigger doll may be stronger and greater, each is equally important to the concept of the whole. We can use our 5 senses to understand our physical selves, but all levels are important in our health and healing, even if we can't tangibly sense them. They work together harmoniously in flow of balance, also known as a fluid state of homeodynamics. Therefore, when one level is out of alignment, a message or symptom is delivered to the corresponding area of the body to attempt to stimulate a readjustment and bring the person back into balance.

Since most conventional medicine targets only the first level, we may never achieve full healing using only low level medical methods. A perfect example – many people who start anti-depressants have a very hard time coming off of them, even long after the initial stressful or traumatic event that precipitated their use is over. Why? Because they may have never sought healing on the emotional or perhaps the unconscious mental level to create balance and resolve of the underlying issues. In this example, the root issue would not be on the first level, so the body may never heal unless they can tap into the third or fourth level of healing.

Another way to think of the levels of healing is like a horse drawn carriage. The carriage is your physical body that is required to take you from point A to B. Without it, you couldn't get anywhere. If you don't take care of it – oil the hinges, replace old boards, fix the tires, and so on – you would be very slow to arrive at your required destination, if at all.

The horses are the emotional body – they are the driving force, the passionate accelerators. They get you moving. They also require blinders, because they can easily steer you off course if they *feel* so compelled. The horses need to be able to stay focused in the direction the driver requires.

The driver, who holds the reins of the horses, is the mental body. He/she is responsible for taking the most logical and efficient path to your destination. The driver is able to steer clear of washed out roads and navigate around detours. For the most part the driver steers unconsciously in auto-pilot, much like when you drive your own car – but when obstacles appear, the conscious mind has to take over.

The energetic body is the connection between all of these things: the carriage, the horses and the driver. It's the language and communication between these elements that keeps the vessel uniform and working harmoniously together – from the reins, to the gears, to the brakes, to the verbal commands. Without connection, the levels remain separate and dissonant.

All of these aspects of a functioning working carriage are important, and work perfectly together… but they are merely parts of you, not who you truly are.

Ask yourself, what is the point of a horse drawn carriage? To take a *passenger* to their destination, from A to B. You are the passenger – all levels of your body including your soul with a purpose and a journey on this earth. The soul harnesses your spiritual essence. Understand that in this view of the body you require each of these levels, but in turn, pathology may lie in each one. This leads us to understand that we must find healing on the right level in order to truly be well.

It is also important to note that the root causes and symptoms we learned about in Part 1, may each have an effect on every one of the healing levels. I will discuss this further in each chapter, but there is not a linear association between the main root causes and the main levels of healing. We are dynamic and complex, so the connection is not always clear-cut – but when we discover all of our roots, the layers of healing required will then become very apparent.

In the chapters that follow we will talk about each of these bodies in detail, as well as the corresponding treatments connected to our root disease. After reading these chapters, my aim is that you will be equipped with the knowledge of where your body needs to heal, and will feel empowered on your path to healing.

SEVEN

First Level: Physical Body

"After all, no one ever hated their own body, but they feed and care for
their body."
~Ephesians 5:29

"To keep the body in good health is a duty, otherwise we shall not be
able to keep our mind strong and clear."
~Buddha

*Eleven-year-old Makayla is a courageous young girl with a spirit of determi-
nation. When she came into my office nearly 2 years ago, she had already
lost all of her hair. It had started twelve months prior with patchy hair loss,
and at that time was rectified by a steroid cream. However, after about eight
months, Makayla started to get larger areas of hair loss that weren't growing
back. She also started feeling fatigued, along with foggy thinking. Shortly
after this she had her thyroid tested, and although the function was normal,
her thyroid antibodies were high. She then proceeded to lose all of her hair
and began to notice poor healing and growth, body temperature dysregulation, and more "allergy-type" symptoms. She also was having more regular
stomach aches, especially after eating sugary or processed foods. Despite the*

complete loss of her hair, she was vibrant and brave, and her mother was just as determined to get answers, which landed them in my office.

Makayla did have some family history of autoimmune disease on her father's side, but neither of her parents reported significant health concerns. She did report she had a serious staph infection at an early age, as well as some recent vaccinations and pesticide exposures from living on an orchard.

This wasn't the first case of alopecia I had treated in a young girl, so I knew we had to get to the bottom of the inflammatory reactive process that was causing her hair to fall out. We tested for food sensitivities, and also put her on a strict gluten and cane sugar-free diet. Even though she didn't have celiac disease according to her blood test, the fact that she was confirmed with Hashimoto's thyroiditis meant being gluten-free was an absolute necessity. In my experience, autoimmune diseases are often rooted in gluten intolerance, chronic toxicity from heavy metals, or chronic infection. When dealing with autoimmune thyroid conditions, I also add in EMF exposure and possibly fluoride toxicity to the list of root causes that we need to examine.

Upon reviewing Makayla's history, it looked as though there were several possible physical root causes that needed to be investigated and ruled out. Her previous significant infection, several toxin exposures through her environment, and her vaccination history could all have been causative agents to her hair loss. These experiences all fall under the physical realm of health because they are actual material things that we can associate with the senses of taste, touch, sight, smell or sound. They are tangible and visible.

The physical body is easiest to understand by reflecting on your relationship to the conventional medical paradigm. Anything that has to do with the physical body is in the material dimension, where we find the structure of elements into matter. Matter consists of what we can see with our eyes, and measure easily and objectively.

In medicine, we can assess the physical body in many ways – from blood, urine, or saliva tests, to skin allergy tests, to physical exams. Medical care also includes a multitude of treatments such as medications, dietary changes, surgery, chiropractic care, herbal medicine, IV therapies, orthomolecular medicine (high dose vitamin therapy), physiotherapy, massage, ozone therapy, stem cell transplants, gene therapy, heavy metal chelation, exercise or aromatherapy, to name a few. That is a huge list and I would bet everyone has experienced at least one of these types of therapies in their lives. These treatments are important, and sometimes all we need. Many times, however, they just scratch the surface, especially for more complicated, persistent and long-term symptoms.

The physical level is where most of our symptoms end up, despite the level of origin. This is because the physical level is directly under the effect of all other levels. It is the lowest level of the body, but no less important. We are most aware of this level, as it is quite literally the foundation sitting under all other levels. It is where physical pain and discomfort lie. The physical body is always present in the now. It doesn't know future or past tense (that is the mind), therefore what you think, you physically feel instantly. This is why your body experiences both actual and imagined symptoms in real time.

Therefore, regardless of what level the imbalance started on, disease often shows up on the physical level. However, like that horse drawn carriage analogy, the physical body does have a finite capacity. It is limited literally by its own physical space. If we push our physical body past its capacity to balance and heal for too long, eventually problems will show up, just like in the example of Lacy in Chapter 6, where her physical body eventually reached burnout.

Although we may be aware that we have an infinite soul's capacity for wellness and healing, the limits to our health are literally only what the physical body can withstand. Remember, this body is the physical vehicle, the carrier of our spirit, and without it we are literally not here on this earth in a physical state. So it is best to keep our body in great condition – not only to feel well, but also to be able to fulfill our individual life purpose.

Let's talk about some of the key root causes to disease that we have discussed, and the corresponding treatments on the physical level:

1) GENETICS:

Until lately, we have had very little ability to influence our "genetic code." There is now new research in this area that is investigating the possibility of gene therapy, where one can turn on or turn off a specific gene. However, it has also been discovered that we do have influence over our own genes, explained through the theory of epigenetics. Meaning the cleaner, happier and more balanced the environment around our cells, the more positive gene expression we can anticipate. This could be as simple as eating a clean, organic diet. In the book, *Eat Right 4 Your Type*, Dr. D'Adamo talks about optimal health and disease prevention being connected to the types of foods eaten. Foods are emphasized in relation to your genetic blood type and geographic heritage. He also suggests that this is particularly imperative for pregnant women, when the fetus' gene selection is even more active.[71] On a physical level this also means keeping a clean body terrain by minimizing inflammation, infections, environmental toxins, nutrient deficiencies and stress, all of which we will discuss further. As you may have already guessed, all of the root causes are interrelated.

2) NUTRIENT DEFICIENCIES:

You must support proper digestion. In my office this is always a three stage process, and everyone requires specific interventions to resolve deficiencies.

I. Stage 1: Remove

a. In a general sense, you must first clean up the gut – take any food allergies out of the diet, identified either by IgG testing, biofeedback testing or elimination diets. It is also important we clean up the diet. Most of us consume way too much sugar, bad fats and processed foods. It will be impossible to heal the gut if you continue eating damaging foods, even if you eliminate your allergies. You don't want to end up reacting to the new foods that replace the allergenic foods.

Eating clean really means eating whole foods, non-GMO and organic, as much as possible. This means avoiding processed food. What is processed? Anything that comes in a box, can or jar required some processing. So be aware of labels. What has been added to that food to get it in that container? How close to its natural form does it now look?

You lose nutrients with any processing, even cooking, so the more whole the food is, the more nutritional quality it has. I also encourage patients to buy local – not only does that support your local community and the environment, but there is less likely to be degradation of nutrients from being shipped long distances away.

And finally, focus on a balanced meal. Most North American diets are high in carbohydrates with a high glycemic index: sugar, starches and grains. They are great for energy, but most of us with sedentary lifestyles will never use all those excess calories. We are actually meant to burn fat for energy, but the more carbs we have available, the more our bodies will preferentially use them over our stored fats, because it's easier for the body to metabolize. Hence when I say eat a balanced meal, I suggest it looks more like the diagram below:

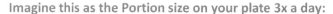

Imagine this as the Portion size on your plate 3x a day:

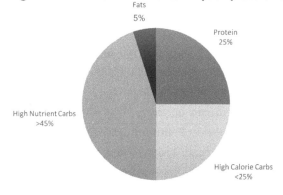

Fats
5%

Protein
25%

High Nutrient Carbs
>45%

High Calorie Carbs
<25%

- Fats (*serving size of your thumbs*): cold pressed vegetable or seed oils, raw nuts, raw seeds, avocados, coconut oil, olives, oily fish
- Protein (*size of your palm including thickness*): meat, poultry, seafood, fish, eggs, legumes, beans, protein powders, hemp seeds, raw nuts, tofu
- High Calorie Carbs (*size of your fist*): breads, cereals, pasta, chips, flours, root vegetables like potatoes and yams, corn, all grains like rice or quinoa, sweets, carrots, peas, fruits like bananas, grapes, mango or pineapple (some in this category are more beneficial than others)
- High Nutrient Carbs (*2 hands cupped together like a bowl*): green leafy vegetables, broccoli, cauliflower, peppers, cucumber, zucchini, celery, (and almost every single vegetable out there), apples, peaches, pears, oranges, grapefruit, berries, lentils.

There has been recent popularity around the macrobiotic, paleolithic, and ketogenic diets for example, and although they each specifically may have benefit for certain people and particular diseases, in general a high nutrient dense diet is always beneficial. The precise caloric breakdown and food choices will depend on an individual's allergies, sensitivities, activity level, blood type, ethics, and food availability.

b. In this first stage, removal, you also want to clear out any infections. Depending on the patient this may be relatively simple, or it can take a very long time. Treatment for infections will be discussed further in this chapter.

c. It's also important at this stage that you support stomach acid. This helps you to prevent infections by killing pathogens. It also assists in nutrient absorption by breaking down food properly. Supportive levels of stomach acid can be fostered by simple means, such as chewing our food properly, limiting fluids with meals, focusing on eating at mealtime (no multi-tasking), and taking 10 deep breaths before eating (to activate the parasympathetic nervous system). We can also assist it with one-quarter teaspoon of apple cider vinegar before meals, traditional bitter blends like Swedish bitters before meals, or Betaine HCL pills. If there is actual damage in the stomach lining or you are already on antacids, this process may take time as you will need to also heal the gut as you regain function. Stomach healers can include deglycerated licorice (DGL), zinc carnosine or mastic gum, to name a few.

II. Stage 2: Repair

a. The second stage in restoring a healthy nutrient balance is to repair – to heal the intestinal lining. In addition to the stomach healers listed above, there are many other digestive healers – like slippery elm, marshmallow root, aloe vera, and L-glutamine. This process typically takes months and requires continued eating of a clean, allergy free diet. Further down the digestive tract, there also may be the need for some colon cleansing at this point in order to heal the entire digestive system. Common remedies I suggest for detox are supplements with dematiaceous earth, bentonite clay, activated charcoal, humic acid, ground flax seeds, psyllium or aloe vera juice. If you are using digestive binders like dematiaceous earth, activated charcoal or bentonite clay, you should be cautious as these remedies can be constipating if used in high quantities or taken without adequate water.

III. Stage 3: Replace

a. The final stage of digestive healing is to restore your digestive flora – ensure your gut (from the mouth/sinus to the anus) is full of healthy bacteria. So much research has been done on microorganisms and their role in chronic diseases. From specific bacterial strains that treat different diseases, to fecal transplants to cure diabetes, this is medically a new frontier. We are only beginning to understand the complexities that the digestive flora "environment" has on our health. Keeping an optimal flora is found to be key. Therefore, maintaining balance by eating a clean, healthy diet is imperative. This concept isn't new, it has just recently begun to be commercialized. As early as the 1900s, researchers like Eli Metchnikoff linked longevity with consuming fermented foods like yogurt.[72]

More recently, there has been a huge movement in the creation and consumption of fermented foods. Eating foods such as kombucha, yogurt, sauerkraut, kimchi and kefir, as well as just taking probiotics regularly, seems to be essential to the digestive tract functioning optimally. Thus, in order to maintain healthy nutrient levels, the flora balance and intestinal integrity are imperative.

Treatments for Nutrient Absorption and Digestive Health:

a) Food Quality
    i)   Eat organic and non-GMO to ensure the highest nutritional value
    ii) Eat local
    iii) Eat raw and fresh foods
    iv) Cook from fresh or frozen for best nutritional quality

b) Absorption
    i)   Chew your food fully
    ii) Eat slowly to allow for proper digestion
    iii) Avoid eating fruit with proteins and starchy carbs which slow digestion down
    iv) Take digestive support like Betaine HCL or ¼ tsp. apple cider vinegar before meals
    v) Take digestive enzymes with meals only if necessary
    vi) Utilize bitters like gentian or Swedish bitters to stimulate digestion

c) Utilization
    i)   Chiropractic, physiotherapy or osteopathic treatments can help with anatomical misalignment which may impede digestive function
    ii) Tissue salts can stimulate mineral utilization in the body (like Ferrum Phos 6X for iron utilization)

3) TOXINS:

This root cause of disease resides largely in the physical level, as we discussed in the multiple examples in the toxicity chapter. Treatment of toxins depends on the type and the area of the body that is affected:

a) Internal Toxins: Endotoxins, also known as toxins from within the body that occur due to normal metabolism and bodily functions, can best be cleared through good hydration. The average person should consume approximately one-third to one-half of their weight in pounds, in ounces of water per day (i.e. a 150-pound person should drink between 50-75 ounces of water a day, that's about 6-9 cups)!

Keep in mind that if you consume caffeinated drinks, that number should go up because they act as a diuretic. So for every cup of coffee, add another two cups of water. Might be easier and more beneficial to reduce coffee intake rather than spend the day in the bathroom! We are approximately 60-70% water so we need it to flush out the system.[73]

Maintaining a good healthy terrain through digesting fermented foods, as well as avoiding GMOs, also helps to reduce our internal toxic burden. We can also take probiotic supplements and avoid antibiotics as much as possible, as well as foods and products that contain them (non-organic meats, antibacterial soaps, etc.).

b) Heavy metals: They accumulate in our system, whether we like it or not.

i) As discussed in Chapter 3, you can avoid some common sources:

- Limit larger fish and most seafood (particularly farmed and canned versions) high in mercury. Smaller fish tend to have the lowest levels like sardines, mackerel and herring.
- Be aware of the toxic burden associated with vaccinations, particularly aluminum and mercury, through avoidance if advisable, or drainage remedies if not.
- Avoid certain cosmetics like long lasting lip sticks with lead or shimmery powders with bismuth.
- Avoid lead based paints or varnishes.
- Wear masks when dealing with old paints, cars or welding.
- Try to avoid fire retardant clothing and furniture.
- Avoid aluminum/tin foils, pots and cans.
- Avoid putting mercury amalgams in your teeth and replace the ones that you already have with a benign composite (seek out a dentist trained in proper SMART technique; use IAOMT as resource).[74]

ii) Chelation removes heavy metals from the body. Once levels are tested and determined using urine provocation tests, it is typically the therapy of choice. Common agents used are EDTA, DMPS or DMSA, some of which are administered through an IV, and others orally. Chelation should always be administered only by a trained and certified physician who is aware of, and monitors, your chronic heavy metal load.

iii) Natural agents or therapies also have evidence of chelating (bonding to and removing) some heavy metals, including: chlorella, liposomal glutathione, cilantro, zeolites, humic acid, alpha lipoic acid, and Far Infrared sauna use.

c) *External toxins*: These toxins enter the body through the mouth, skin, and lungs, and should be avoided to the best of our ability. The following practices will help you avoid ingesting toxins:

i) Mouth:

(1) Eat an organic diet as much as possible – at the very least avoid the dirty dozen: strawberries, spinach, nectarines, apples, peaches, pears, cherries, grapes, celery, tomatoes, sweet bell peppers and potatoes (check out www.ewg.org). [75]

(2) Eat GMO-free foods – read labels, as it is not required by law to declare GMOs! Look for the voluntary Non-GMO or Certified Organic labels (it's your only way to guarantee it is GMO-free). Top GMO foods to avoid: corn, soy, cottonseed oil, beet sugar, alfalfa, canola, dairy and beef (from cows fed GMO grains), Hawaiian papaya, aspartame, zucchini, yellow squash and infant formulas.

(3) Avoid cooking foods at high heats, such as in frying or charbroiling, where toxic carcinogens can form.

(4) Choose raw and even sprouted foods more often, especially in warmer months: fruits, vegetables, nuts and seeds.

(5) When cooking foods, prepare at lower temperatures with ceramics, stoneware, glass or even better, high grade stainless steel like

Saladmaster cookware. These will leach the least amount of toxic chemicals or heavy metals into your foods. Most regular stainless steel pots will leach their metal cores, most commonly aluminum, under high heats into your food. Avoid non-stick surfaces, as this coating will also leach into your foods when cooking.

(6) Store your food in glass, not plastic.

(7) Never use plastic of any grade in the microwave (or avoid it altogether)!

(8) Try to avoid purchasing foods in cans or in juice box tetra packs as they are lined with BPA plastics.

(9) Wash your dishes using a chemical free, earth friendly dish or dishwasher soap.

(10) Filter your drinking water. I am a big believer in utilizing the water we already have, without purchasing bottled water at a huge expense for you and the plastic waste to the environment. However, I also believe most of us have contaminated water, as many drinking water sources contain chlorine, fluoride, lead, uranium, cesium and thallium, as well as pesticides, herbicides, and medications from urinary excretion – so filtration is ideal.[76] Spring water is great in theory, but most of us don't have a spring of fresh glacier water in our backyard. I personally use a reverse osmosis *remineralized* water system. The key here being that the RO water is remineralized: i.e. it has a system that replaces the good filtered minerals as well as removing the harmful elements. There are also various alkalinisation systems on the market, but be sure to check if they will also filter the water first. Carbon filters, like those included on a fridge water system, are better than nothing but may not take out the smaller particles such as environmental toxins or recirculated pharmaceuticals.

ii) Lungs:

(1) Invest in a good quality air purifier, either for your entire house or

a single room (most important to use in your bedroom).

(2) Change or clean your air filters regularly on your furnace and air conditioning unit.

(3) Avoid or limit exposure to areas of smoke and chemical spraying (e.g. on farms, orchards or golf courses) as much as possible.

(4) Wear a mask at work if using hazardous chemicals (always)!

(5) Make sure your area is well ventilated if working with paints, perfumes, glues or cleaning products, and protect your lungs and skin from contact.

iii) Skin:

(1) If you wouldn't put it in your mouth, don't put it on your skin! It's going to get inside your body eventually. Be sure the ingredients are familiar and organic if possible.

(2) Avoid: parabens, sodium laurel sulphate, oxybenzone, octinoxate, retinyl palmitate, triclosan, propylene glycol, phthalates, toluene, formaldehyde, mineral oils or petroleum products (any by-products harvested from oil and gas industry). Read labels as these are in many products (particularly in personal hygiene products) – they are all toxic to the body.

(3) Avoid cosmetics, perfumes and personal hygiene products with synthetic dyes and additives. Go to safecosmetics.org or goodguide.com to check out your product's safety.

(4) Switch over to natural based cleaners like vinegar, essential oils and baking soda whenever possible; you can even try silver lined cloths for a chemical free cleaning, like Norwex.

(5) Avoid chemical based detergents, dry cleaning chemicals, fabric softeners and dryer sheets. These may be one of the worst toxic exposures to the skin as we are in constant contact all day long. Many skin irritations and rashes are simply due to these chemicals. There are many natural effective laundry cleaners on the market.

Methods to support our organs in detoxification (all products and treatments must be used under the guidance of a trained professional for appropriate timing and dosage):

(1) **Liver and Gallbladder**:
   (a) Herbs: greater celandine, turmeric, milk thistle, yellow dock, garlic, artichoke, dandelion root
   (b) Supplements: SAMe, N-Acetyl cysteine, vitamin C, vitamin A, B vitamins: particularly B12, B9 and B6, calcium d-glucarate
   (c) Treatments: castor oil packs, hydrotherapy, liver/gallbladder flushes, coffee enemas, grapefruit, coffee, garlic and onions, lemon

(2) **Blood and Lymphatics**:
   (a) Herbs: cleavers, red clover, burdock, manjistha, bupleurum, rehmannia
   (b) Treatments: lymphatic massage, dry skin brushing, exercise, Major Auto Hemo Ozone therapy, rebounders, lemon water, osteopathy

(3) **Brain**:
   (a) Herbs: parsley, cilantro, gingko, guta kola, turmeric, yarrow
   (b) Supplements: liposomal glutathione, alpha lipoic acid, chlorella, methyl-B12, selenium, Co Q10
   (c) Treatments: cranial sacral therapy, chiropractic, osteopathy, ozone therapy

(4) **Skin**:
   (a) Treatments: dry skin brushing, hot/cold showers, hydrotherapy, mineral salt baths, peat or clay masks, infrared saunas

(5) **Colon**:
   (a) Herbs: cascara, slippery elm, turkey rhubarb, aloe vera, psyllium
   (b) Supplements: humic acid, flax seeds, bentonite clay, dematiaceous earth, activated charcoal, calcium D-glucarate
   (c) Treatments: colonics, enemas, rectal ozone

(6) **Kidneys**:
   (a) Herbs: nettles, dandelion leaf, goldenrod, solidago, hydrangea root
   (b) Treatments: hydration! (ideally 1/3-1/2 of your body weight [in pounds converted to ounces]), electrolyte mixes

One of my primary roles in supporting patients through detoxification is to determine if a cleanse is warranted, and if so, the appropriate time and method. If cleanses are not done well or are too aggressive, people often feel worse, not better! I'm not a huge advocate of most generic commercial cleanses from the health food store, as we are all individual in our needs and requirements. Hence, until you have a good handle on how a cleanse will work best for you, start with the basic lifestyle changes mentioned above, then seek guidance to create a detox plan most appropriate for you.

4) INFECTIONS:

When the root cause is infections, we need to identify what they are, and then medicinally attack them with the right effective agents. This should be done with a qualified practitioner. Common effective remedies include:

i) Parasitic:

(1) Herbals: black walnut, artemisinin extract, wormwood, garlic, cloves, olive leaf, mimosa putica, inula, cinchona

(2) Medications: biltricide®, vermox™, pyrantil pamoate, albenza®, ivermectin (if available)

ii) Fungal:

(1) Herbals: p'au darco, grapefruit seed extract, garlic, capryllic acid, berberine alkaloids, olive leaf, tea tree, reishi mushroom

(2) Medications: nystatin, fluconazole, ketoconazole, metronidazole

iii) Bacterial:

(1) Herbals: berberine alkaloids, garlic, golden seal, echinacea, Oregon grape, cat's claw, banderol, cumanda, yarrow, lomanteum, inula, houttuynia, olive leaf, stevia, bee propolis

(2) Medications: several antibiotics (although there hasn't been a new class of antibiotics produced in over 30 years!) – penicillins, ciprofloxacin, biaxin™, erythromycin, cefuroxine, rifampin, minocycline, doxycycline are some examples

iii) Viral:

(1) Herbals: astragalus, boneset, echinacea, garlic, reishi mushroom, oregano oil, elderberry, olive leaf

(2) Medications: acyclovir and similar medicines

iv) Biofilms:

(1) Herbals: enzymes, nattokinase, lumbrokinase, berberine, silicea tissue salts, stevia, serrapeptase, apple cider vinegar, garlic

(2) Medications or synthetics heparin, EDTA, xylitol

(3) Treatments: neural therapy

We started this chapter by learning about Makayla's case, where she was looking for a cause for her hair loss. We started digging into all of the relevant root causes of disease. We removed the easy ones first: EMFs by turning things off and wearing a grounder, changing to a non-fluorinated toothpaste (fluoride competes with iodine in the thyroid) and incorporating a gluten-free diet (an extremely common inflammatory food in autoimmune disease). We also added in some key nutrients like B vitamins and minerals to address nutrient deficiencies.

We then began to plug away at toxicity and infections. The first area that we addressed was her heavy metal exposure, starting with a simple protocol of liposomal glutathione and chlorella, which are natural chelators. I then started to treat both a parasite that was confirmed on a stool sample, and bacteria. Within a few short months Makayla started to notice patchy hair growth. Her mother supported her to continue to radically change her diet to GMO free and organic, including more juicing. Despite all the peer pressures that kids can face, Makayla stuck to the plan. She continued to see hair growth. She even started to notice growth spurts and increased energy, and her stomach pains went away.

A year after we started she had a full head of hair – some patchy spots, but several inches in length in some areas as well. She was almost ready for a haircut. Even her alopecia community, for which she was an advocate and fundraiser, was amazed. We continued to work on clearing heavy metals and layers of infections, with the ultimate goal of resetting her immune system.

As we have continued on, Makayla's immune system is still the primary focus; if we stray off the path or she has some new toxin exposures, it tends to show up in resumed hair loss. She may never be able to eat gluten, as I feel this food is a direct inflammatory trigger for her, but living a full, healthy, balanced life is a much greater reward. We are peeling through the layers and getting closer and closer to immune stability. She is a leader for her generation, gaining courage and knowledge from her experience. The world our children are growing up in is very different than in previous generations. They will have to become advocates for prevention and health as the environment becomes increasingly toxic, adulterated and over stimulating. Every child that has a health success story today, is ultimately an advocate for a new movement of health for tomorrow. These children are inspirational and the purest sense of humanity that we can see. It's a privilege to work with these kids, as they are so open to the healing process.

Makayla's example is a clear case of healing occurring primarily on the physical level, since that was where the roots lay. In this case we dealt with toxicity, chronic infection, food allergies, nutrient deficiencies and electromagnetic frequencies. The very fact that she noticed the change in her symptoms from just these types of interventions confirms that the healing required was primarily in the physical body. Some cases resolve in this way, but others, even with the same symptoms, do not – they require a deeper level of healing.

5) STRESS:

You always feel stress on a physical level, regardless of the cause, because the fight or flight response of stress directly affects the body's ability to function. Longer term, stress will affect your body digestively, reproductively, immunologically and hormonally. The more you can seek to achieve a balanced state, the better.

If you have experienced high and chronic stress, you will need to support the body on a physical level by restoring adrenal function – to build the adrenal glands back up to a normal functioning status. This could involve resolving nutrient deficiencies, commonly B5, B6, B12, magnesium and vitamin C. This could also mean using herbs like ashwaganda, rhodiola, relora, ginseng and licorice (and ideally, one would only ever use stimulating herbs like panax ginseng, licorice, ephedra or caffeine when the adrenals are already in a nutritionally optimal place).

I find patients often like the feeling of stimulants and may get addicted to them – but I remind them that in the long run, caffeine is running down their adrenal function faster. People experiencing chronic stress should avoid stimulating herbs like caffeine, licorice and ginseng, and stick to toners like rhodiola and holy basil.

Finally, adrenal function can be supported by adrenal glandulars from porcine or bovine sources, although these are amongst the stronger supplementations and should only be used short term, under the care of a practitioner. The adrenal glands may experience dysfunction in two ways as we discussed previously:

a) **Hyperadrenism:** In this case, we want to bring the cortisol down from a chronic hyperstimulated state.

  i) Supplements: phosphatidylserine, L-theanine, avena sativa (oat straw), melissa officinalis (lemon balm), kava, melatonin

  ii) Treatments: activate the parasympathetic via deep breathing, prayer, meditation, sleeping or relaxation

b) **Hypoadrenism:** In this case, cortisol is low and we want to support the adrenal glands to produce cortisol more efficiently.

  i) Supplements: ashwaganda, holy basil, rhodiola, roseola, licorice, Siberian ginseng, B vitamins, magnesium, vitamin C

  ii) Treatments: massage, deep breathing, medications like Cortef® or adrenal glandulars (only to be used under physician prescription and care), reduction of exercise intensity (important as exercise is a form of stress – low to moderate intensity will serve your adrenals and help build your exercise tolerance)

Sleep and rest are always effective combatants to stress – as are any activities that instill gentle relaxation like meditation, yin yoga, prayer or just play. Play is often highly overlooked, and patients often laugh when I "prescribe" it to them. Sometimes we actually have to figure out what play even means to us again. Kids can be excellent teachers in this department. One of my favorite "play" activities after a long day is a spontaneous dance party with my daughters in the living room – we move the coffee table, turn the music up loud and let loose! These activities are applicable to both the hyperadrenal and hypoadrenal state because both are on the same continuum, the latter is just literally further down the burnout trail.

c) **Adrenal Fatigue:** In this state the person is no longer functioning in a normal capacity. They are often gripped with chronic inflammation in some area of the body and chronic fatigue. These patients typically have several root causes, but from a stress perspective it is important to just support, not stimulate the adrenals, or they will in fact prolong the recovery. This is where adrenal glandular support is more regularly used by practitioners. Patients with adrenal fatigue also benefit from mitochondrial support: CoQ10, d-ribose, L-carnitine, grapeseed extract, magnesium, alpha lipoic acid or glutathione support. Other than the mitochondrial support, supplementation is going to be very similar to that used for the hypoadrenal state, just likely stronger and for a longer period of time.

In the adrenal fatigue state, there are often several areas in the body that are affected. Therefore, treatment would typically involve more systems, often thyroid support, hormonal support, digestive support and infection clearing. Although adrenal support is the foundation, more areas will need to be addressed in this multisystem approach.

Overall, no matter what the disease, holistic healing always addresses the whole person, not just one body area or level.

Summary

As you can see, there are many ways in which we can address the root causes of the physical body. This can include many types of treatment such as herbal remedies, nutrient support, physical therapies, and at times where appropriate, even pharmaceutical drugs. Although the cause of the disease may not lie in the physical level, it is very important to support and heal the physical body regardless. We are not meant to ignore a symptom; it is a messenger. We do have to keep our physical carriage in great shape to keep us moving forward in life!

It is also vital to remember – just because we experience a physical symptom, it does *not* mean the root is only physical. The physical level is the most basic, primal level of self, and symptoms on this level are often a last ditch effort for your body to address issues that have not been dealt with on a deeper level. It's not a coincidence that physical signs have a more effective way of getting our attention. This is especially true if we are more apt to ignore or be disassociated from our inner levels of self, consciously or unconsciously. So understand, if your symptoms do not resolve with physical medicine, or are only *controlled* by continuous use of physical medicine (and cannot be explained by a permanent physical limitation like an accident or disability), then you may not have reached the right level of healing yet. We need to go deeper into your inner self to find where that healing may dwell. There are answers. The body is speaking. The symptom always has meaning. We just need to hear it.

EIGHT

Second Level: Energetic Body

"There has been a revolution in how we perceive the body. What appears to be an object, a three-dimensional anatomical structure, is actually a process, a constant flow of energy and information."
~Deepak Chopra

Tanya, at age thirty-three, had been suffering from chronic diffuse pain all over her body for years. By the time she found herself in my office, although it caused her significant limitations in her work capacity and regretful isola-tion socially, she had all but succumbed to her plight in life, to always feeling physical pain. The pain would migrate from joint to limb, with no real pattern, and it exhausted her. She didn't seem to know a definitive time when it started, but thought that overall it was getting worse. Her initial intake revealed that she did suffer physical and emotional abuse at a very young age, but her memories were foggy, and she didn't remember much detail. She had left home at a fairly young age, and preferred to leave the past, just as that, the past. She felt like she had dealt with the impact of the abuse, despite the fact that she wasn't able to stay in an intimate committed relationship throughout her life, preferring to stay well within her comfort zone. Upon testing her in the office with biofeedback techniques, I determined she had interference field or energetic block in her system that was stopping her body's self-regulation mechanisms. Biofeedback can utilize several methods, as stated previously in Chapter 4 of this book, but the premise of the testing is to energetically challenge the autonomic nervous system through different filters, testers or remedies to determine what stresses the system, and consequently how the body needs to be supported.

The Energetic Body, or second level, is quite literally where the energetic pulse of our human existence resides. It is the vitality that flows through our body. In homeopathy it is called our Vital Force, in Asian medicine it is called Chi or Qi, for Yogis it's prana, and Indian cultures may refer to it as Shakti. Some people even feel that they can see a person's life force by the auras that surround them.

Your energetic body connects every level of self (physical, emotional, mental) to create your whole being. We are energy, because we are made of molecules of energy. When you look at a cell under a microscope, it is comprised of different proteins, derived from different molecules, fashioned from a collection of atoms, formed by their corresponding protons, neutrons and electrons – which are really just space and energy. The movement of these tiny particles of substance, and their interaction with other substances makes up all the different objects of matter we see today! How these molecules are put together makes each of us, and every living thing, who we are. Ironically, looking at outer space is very much like looking into our inner space.

The laws of physics study the correlation of energy and mass, energy waves, force and time. This is represented in the human body in our physiology... or rather, in how the body works. So as you can see, the energetic body is not a foreign concept –maybe just something you haven't thought about in the context of your health. When we talk about how the body works, we're talking about its function, which requires energy.

Every life form contains energy within – you could say energy is the Life Force that keeps the spiritual and physical bodies connected.

When we eat food, we harness the life force from plants or animals to replenish our own, as we have expelled ours in heat or movement or metabolism. As explained by the laws of physics, energy is neither created nor destroyed, just transferred from one form to another. A plant has to harness and store the sunlight's energy, so when we eat plants, we form the energy molecules that are needed to perform our vital life functions. Our bodies then transform this energy into another state – such as movement, sound, vibration or light. Since we are energetic beings, we are constantly interacting with our environment to transform energy into versions that we require for the very essence of life. The nature of this flow of energy corresponds to the nature of the flow we see in and around ourselves. Hence it is imperative to allow the energy to flow properly in the body to be able to stay connected and in alignment with our physical bodies and emotional/mental/spiritual bodies. Energy is the segue between the levels.

In Western Medicine, energy is associated with our nervous system, a network of electrical wires that communicate in the body through the conductivity of an electrical pulse that transports energy. This system operates so quickly that we have no cognition of anything occurring. It regulates every movement, every autonomic function, every reflex, every impulse.

The majority of conventional testing methods today assess our biochemistry for what are considered to be abnormalities – blood work being one common example. These types of tests look only at the physical level, they will not show function. Energetic functional tests include methods like biofeedback testing, Reba or Vega machines, auricular testing, Chinese pulses, cranial sacral assessments, thermograms, X-rays, MRI's, EKG's, EEG, EAV, Kirland photography and even ultrasound.

Our energy flows through us like a river, whether we call it nerves, meridians or chakras. How well it flows determines our health on this level. When the flow is blocked, some area in the body downstream is affected. This is the whole premise of Chinese medicine – opening up the meridians and restoring proper flow in the body so nothing is in excess (before the block) or deficiency (after the block). The process of yoga and meditation can also be therapies to attempt to open up and move energy in the body to stimulate flow.

How do you know if your energy is blocked? Sometimes people literally say they "feel blocked," even if they don't really know what that means. I have also heard people in my office say, "Nothing seems to change my health," or "Nothing works," or "Treatments never last for me." Sometimes, they'll describe their own case as "difficult or challenging." These experiences could certainly indicate a block.

Other times, patients describe experiencing a lot of neurological symptoms like numbness, dizziness, pain or tremors – or even cognitive symptoms like anxiety, memory loss, tics or confusion. In these cases, the nervous system could be experiencing physical symptoms from a number of causes – a concussion, injury, EMF exposure, surgery or a trauma, for example.

In addition, you may also see a physical symptom show up in one area of the body that is connected to a completely different area of physical trauma (which again, may have a number of causes such as a surgery, root canal, accident or an injury). When I say connected, I am referring to the energetic connections in the body as defined in such methods as reflexology or auricular acupuncture. These approaches are based on the principle of one area in the body – the feet, hands or ears, for example – affecting the energy in another area of the body.

There are actually full maps of all of our organs and systems represented on all sorts of body parts: the feet, the hands, the ear, the face and even the teeth! Wow, we are amazing beings. This brings me to our previous case study of Hugh who had his more than thirty year old front root canal removed, and then found that the numbness in his foot went away and discomfort in his hip improved (see Chapter 4). The only way to understand this result is through the explanation of energetic connection between the body parts and the nerves, meridians or Chakras.

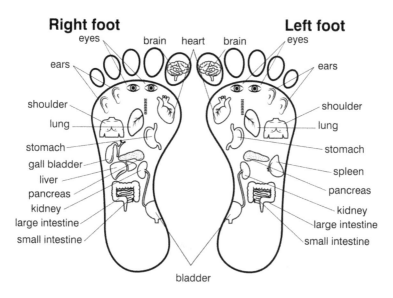

The term interference fields is used to literally refer to that block in the energy flow. Interference fields can be caused by many circumstances including infections, physical trauma, emotional trauma or chemical irritation. Skin and tissue scars are very common interference fields. It's literally like putting a dam of chaotic connective tissue in the river of energetic flow! Yet, not all scars are interference fields. Based on my experience over the years, I believe that the scars that become energy blocks in the body are holding or harnessing a trauma that was associated with the scars at the time of the occurrence – even if the trauma didn't directly result in the scar. For example, I sometimes find the tiniest little scars can be significant, and when treated, patients can feel a huge emotional release. This might show up in a circumstance cutting their finger while chopping vegetables, all the while they were thinking about the divorce they were going through or the death of a loved one. Still, it is much more common that direct scars cause an energetic block – such as in Tanya's case below, where many of the scars were from her childhood physical abuse.

Tanya's physical exam revealed several old scars from her childhood, some from falls or cuts, others from minor injuries she likely sustained at the hand of her father. I explained to her how neural therapy was a very specific therapy that helps to open up blocks in the body on the energetic level, and that it has been used for decades throughout Europe. It's a very safe needle technique that can be used in an area with a scar. It resets the parts of the neurological system that are associated with an area of the body containing the scar.

During the injection treatment of these superficial scars, Tanya began to experience specific memory recalls from her past and was overcome by emotion. (I can attest that this is a common reaction, because of the very nature that the scars are holding emotional memory to traumatic events.) I figured she had a good treatment, and this experience was a great sign of an emotional release. Once she felt relaxed again, I asked her to be kind to herself over the next few days, drink a lot of water to allow for flushing, and check back in a few weeks.

Sure enough, three weeks later, when she returned from her single neural therapy session, she was completely pain free. And when I saw her again six months later, she still reported feeling no pain. Wow! Even I was shocked! I knew the power of this healing modality and had seen many amazing results with neural therapy, but never a complete resolve of debilitating chronic symptoms. Her root trauma was completely buried in the energetic level!

A common type of scar that I treat in my practice is a C-section scar, as often the circumstances that led to the C-section were traumatic for the mother. These scars cross the lower abdomen where about four significant Chinese meridians flow. The reproductive area may also have scars from a past surgery or trauma in the pelvis. They may be external or internal (also known as an adhesion). These scars may be from ruptured cysts, endometriosis, abuse, abortions, episiotomies, tubal ligations, ectopic pregnancies and so on. They can also be associated with female health issues, like dyspareunia or painful intercourse, inability to achieve climax, ovarian cysts, recurrent infections, hormone imbalances, prolapse, incontinence and even infertility. I have treated literally hundreds of cases where once the energetic level of the scar is addressed, there is a dramatic shift or even total resolution in healing. Neural therapy is probably one of my most effective treatment therapies for infertility, as energetic blocks in the reproductive area are so commonly connected. This is likely one of the reasons acupuncture is so commonly used to support fertility as well.

Electromagnetic frequencies or EMFs also fall into the energetic level of healing, as they quite literally are energy fields. EMFs are a form of radiation that can influence and damage energy flow in the body, much like their stronger counterparts, X-rays and gamma rays. Hopefully, since learning about this topic in Chapter 5, you understand exactly what EMFs do to our bodies. They disrupt our energy flow, and if we are exposed on a consistent basis, they may literally create an energetic scar. Think about when you use your cordless phone or cell phone on the same ear over and over again. What is that doing to the energy flow in your head or any meridians it may pass?

THERAPIES FOR THE ENERGETIC BODY:

1. Acupuncture and Acupressure Points: This ancient Asian Medicine has been around for thousands of years. The early practitioners, over centuries, located specific areas in the body where the meridian energy flow was close enough to the surface of the skin that it could be tapped into and influenced through needles. This type of medicine discovered the path for each meridian and corresponding "points" of access that were connected to an organ in the body. Therefore, the needles could stimulate or suppress a meridian area to achieve the desired balance in the body. Traditional acupuncture uses these principles, looking to influence the body's Qi energy.

A great example of the philosophy of meridian energy flow at work in modern medicine is the use of Sea-Bands® for motion sickness. These are literally based on Asian medicine, as they work by creating acupressure on the pericardium 6 point, a well-known anti-nausea point. There are literally over 400 acupuncture points that are used to shift the body's flow of energy. Shiatsu massage is another technique that uses the same principles but works simply with pressure on the points rather than needles.

Note that some modern use of needles for localized pain relief, for example, by physiotherapists or other practitioners, differ from the description above. These practitioners are more likely working with a localized neurological involvement to attempt to create a different sensory signal in the body (i.e. to stop pain), than necessarily addressing the whole-body connection. IMS or intramuscular stimulation is another type of needling technique for pain and trigger points, which works more on the physical layer of tissue breakdown and pain management, rather than the energetic level.

2. Neural Therapy: The technique of neural therapy has been around since 1925, when it was first used by the Huneke brothers. It is based on the theory that trauma of all types, like scars or injuries, can produce long-standing disturbances in the electrochemical function of tissues. Its usage is designed to specifically penetrate the areas of interference that are present. Neural therapy works on the nervous system to affect the "interaction between the environment and organism." Or in other words, the "organism is an open system which constantly interacts and exchanges matter/energy with the environment."[77] The nervous system mediates this interaction. Therefore, when neural therapy directly affects the nervous system's regulatory functions, it is dealing with the interface between our bodies and our environment. More specifically, neural therapy has several effects: it increases blood profusion to the area, increases regulation and plasticity of the nervous system, disrupts the pain feedback loops and induces self-regulation or communication in the previously blocked body area.

Neural therapy is an injection technique with the main ingredient being procaine, a mild anesthetic, that primarily serves as an abundant source of potassium ions. This is why we get the initial anesthetic effect of numbness – then, if the injection is done correctly and successfully, it can often instantly and permanently resolve a chronic long standing issue – providing the root lies on the energetic level of healing, as seen in Tanya's case. She felt she had emotionally cleared the trauma, but it was still locked up in the cellular memory and needed to be released energetically.

> **NOTE:** *Neural therapy is very different from injections of drugs like cortisone or Botox into tissues or joints, performed most commonly by your medical doctor, and should not be confused. These injections are physical treatments where the injected medicine is designed to mask or block the pain and interfere with the processes in the body, not regulate them.*

3. Reflexology: This technique is very similar in essence to acupuncture, but the whole energetic body is represented on our feet (see diagram above). It can also be mapped out on the hand or the ear. In this technique, manual pressure is applied to areas of the foot that show imbalance or pain, which correspond to different organs or tissues in the body. It's a simple technique to stimulate energy flow to distinctive areas in the body.

4. Reiki or Touch Therapies: This therapy was developed in Japan, with the intention of moving Ki or life force, helping to shift blockages, and raising the person's overall energetic vitality. Reiki or touch therapy is done through subtle movement over the body in places where the energetic flow resides. Often the practitioner doesn't need to physically touch the patient to influence the energy flow. Like acupuncture, the practitioner is attempting to restore flow in the body.

5. Cranial Sacral Therapy: This is a type of gentle bodywork that adjusts the membranes, tissues and fluids in the brain and spine. The practitioners sense the flow of the cerebral spinal fluid to determine where minor adjustments are to be made to improve the rhythm and flow. They then use slight pressure to give a gentle manipulation to the appropriate area.

6. Radiation: This therapy has been used as a healing modality for cancer for nearly a century and is a very intense form of X-ray energy. It is used to treat a cancerous area by damaging the cellular DNA so that the cancer cell cannot replicate. It therefore can reduce tumour size, slow growth or relieve symptoms. However, it often leaves some collateral damage, so to speak, to the surrounding tissues, as it is often difficult, if not impossible, to completely isolate the exposure to a single targeted abnormal tissue. The use of tattoos and small radiation seeds have helped to localize the treatments more specifically.

7. Yoga: Traditional Hatha yoga is about linking movement and breath to move Shakti energy around the body. However, this would have only been one element in the teachings of yoga traditionally. In modern times the holistic health concept may be lost by the average yoga fitness class, like in Bikram or Ashtanga yoga. Still, the idea of creating a peaceful meditative state with precise movement is about creating a space for the connection to your energetic body.

8. Tai Chi or Qi Gong: Although these traditional practices are different, they have very similar purposes and are just different in execution. Much like yoga, these exercises are about moving your Qi or life force around in the body. They also combine gentle movement, breath meditation and martial arts to enhance overall well-being and health. They move slowly to invigorate relaxation and flow.

9. EMF Treatments: Avoidance is always the best solution; however, acknowledging that this type of technology or our dependence on it will likely not change any time soon, we need to reduce our exposures. As reported by *The 2007 BioInitiative Report*, the existing standards for public safety are completely inadequate to protect your health.[78]

So we must take it into our own hands:

- Turn off Wi-Fi at night
- Turn off cell phone at night or use airplane mode
- Use speaker phone or corded hands-free ear piece
- Install an electrical kill switch in your bedroom, to stop all electrical input
- No electrical equipment, like clocks, radios, diffusers, etc. by your head when sleeping
- Avoid being by power lines for long periods
- Test your home and work environment with an EMF reader
- Avoid seafood and fish from contaminated areas
- Consume spirulina and chlorella
- Take iodine supplementation or consume seaweeds regularly
- Take sea salt and baking soda baths to eliminate radiation exposures
- Take bentonite clay and use in baths

Some of the above may be particularly challenging – for example, when someone is living close to a large power line or a power station, this is not an easy fix. Or perhaps their livelihoods are dependent on consistent use of Wi-Fi and electrical devices. While it may not be possible to totally mitigate EMF exposures that are beyond our control, I do believe the more that we neutralize our energy exposures the better; grounding mats or neutralizing plugs may be effective. These devices give an outlet for excess electrons (grounding you, much like the earth does). I believe the concern with commercial EMF absorbers for your devices is that they will eventually become saturated, deeming them no longer effective, with no real way of knowing exactly when that is. As well, the EMF blockers you put on your devices may reduce their effectiveness, which defeats the purpose of the device use. However, reducing exposure to EMF in ways that are possible for you is still the best advice.

Summary

As we begin to understand on what level our bodies require healing, we can see why some people find healing from certain techniques and not others. There is no universal fix-all method, even for the exact same disease or symptom that someone else is experiencing. We may need to heal many levels of self. This is why for some participating in yoga or Tai Chi transforms their lives, whereas others find acupuncture takes away their pain, or neural therapy shifts their migraines, but these techniques may not work for everyone. For the patients experiencing success with these methods, their root was located in the energetic body.

Sometimes healing needs to occur on several levels, and each layer is a necessary piece to the puzzle. Seeing the whole picture is an evolution. This is also why often, we must move deeper into the body's planes to reveal the next relevant level of healing. As you are moving further into this book, you can begin to connect all the pieces as to why health is so multifaceted and holistic. The more you tune into your own body, the more you can discover all the levels that need to be addressed. Part of the courageous cure is just committing to the journey, then letting each step be revealed.

NINE

Third Level: Emotional Body

"We must turn to nature itself, to the observations of the body in
health and disease to learn the truth."
~Hippocrates

*When Robyn came into my life over twelve years ago, her world was in
complete disarray. She lived a life of immediate gratification and debauchery
in one form or another, in order to combat years of a sense of overriding
shame and unworthiness. When I first met my husband's sister, I knew she
had a kind heart but was completely lost. As she was becoming a new family
member to me, I certainly didn't feel it was my place to help her get on track.
Nor did I wish to, as I learned early on in my career never to offer help until
it's asked for, especially with family. My husband and I just did our best to be
able to include her in our lives and support her when we could. She became
pregnant with her long-time boyfriend at the time, which she would go on to
say saved her life.*

*She quickly decided to stop drugs and alcohol and focus on becoming a
parent. She courageously left her unhealthy relationship, went back to school
to get a stable job as a care aide, and took on the role of a single parent. She
did the best she could, and she loved her daughter very much. However, as the*

years went on, she still slipped here and there, until eventually she had two sides to her life – one that worked and was a mom, and one that was still looking for the next thing that would bring her comfort and an escape. Her heart and desire to speak into others with inspiration was incredible, but she could never quite see her own potential and worth. She continued to juggle this inconsistent life, trying so hard to keep it all together. Unfortunately, her poor coping methods led to frequent moves, a series of unsuccessful relationships, and a lack of reliability. I can remember several times getting together for a visit, and as soon as the kids were in bed, she would head out to the local bar to meet up with some friends. She was good at keeping her "other life" away from her family, but we knew things weren't all roses. It wasn't until she hit what she refers to her rock bottom, waking up on the floor to her daughter after a drug binge, that she decided to take charge of her life. No more excuses.

Robyn became aware that she needed to take charge and make changes in her life. She decided to try to discover the root of her feelings, to figure out what was perpetuating these destructive behaviours in her life. She was addressing her third level of healing, Emotional Body. Health at this level addresses how we are feeling and is connected to what we perceive. Many of us don't stop long enough to ask ourselves how we are feeling, let alone know how to define or express the emotions. Therefore, much of the healing on this level comes from just setting an intention to notice what we are feeling, and then we can figure out how to express these emotions. This is where we find value in traditional psychology and counselling therapies.

Even if we don't always focus on what we are feeling, at some level we know that the emotions are there. It's important to understand that the emotions are an important *part* of us, like the physical body, but the feelings themselves are not the whole story of who we are. They are necessary to navigate and live this life but they don't define us. They just give us momentum and are a reference to what our circumstances are. Rather, we are defined by who we choose to be in each and every moment, and how our behavior reflects our feelings.

Still, many of us feel we *are* our emotions. How many people label themselves as "depressed" if they are having frequent feelings of sadness? Or define themselves as anxious for having uncontrollable, worrisome thoughts? We are not those things – we may be having those thoughts or emotions, but we are not *defined* by them. How we label something can have just as much power over us as the symptom itself.

Emotions are the driving force in the body. The horses in our carriage analogy. If we didn't have emotions, our experience of the world would be very different –disconnected, mundane, stagnant even. Emotions give us a reference or an awareness of *how* we connect with the world around us. How objects, situations, people and events make us feel, gives us large cues to whether they are something we want to have in our lives or not.

Emotions are not meant to be held onto, but rather experienced and then let go. They come on in an instant – registered, felt and then released. For example, when someone tells you a joke, how long does it take for you to laugh? Instantly. And how long do you laugh for? Well, that might depend on the quality of the joke, and maybe even your mood that day, but often the laughter leaves as quickly as it came, and then you're on to the next thing. Well, all emotions are created to be this sort of passing experience. A signal of the connection to our environment... fearful, uneasy, angry – or relaxing, warm, loving and so on.

We naturally want to draw ourselves towards positive feelings – for example, joy, happiness, bliss, lust or connection. These drive us forward to engage more in the circumstances that created these positive feelings. For example, if we feel accepted, loved and connected in a relationship, we will likely want to engage and commit more to that relationship. Conversely, when we feel hurt, rejected, disappointed or ashamed in a relationship, we will be more likely to disengage or even leave.

Emotions are the driving force propelling us in our life, moving us forward with passion and excitement, and equally moving us away from aggravation or pain. These emotions are helpful in determining what to attract and avoid in the moment – however, they can also be all consuming if we give them too much emphasis or even resistance.

Emphasis

In the case of emphasis, let's say that you have a fear of public speaking. You then always avoid this situation, as your mind is convinced it will inevitably end in humiliation. Yet, what if that promotion at work that you've been really wanting requires you to do some public speaking? Is that experience of fear serving you or actually limiting you? Although fear is a God given emotion to keep us out of danger, it can often just keep us limited and stuck, as most fears are based on a *personal* truth, assumption or belief. For example, walking into a lion's den could very well induce fear, and probably even a healthy fear in order to keep you out of danger. However, if no one ever told you that lions were dangerous, or maybe you worked in a zoo, perhaps you wouldn't mind.

Either way it's important to recognize the emotion, but then really decipher where it is coming from. Remember, it is a construct of your mind, attempting to give context to your surroundings. Since how we define our fears is based on our past experiences, belief systems, assumptions, biases, motivations, and so on, the emotion, although real, may not always be in your best interest. Feelings can often masquerade as truth. As in our example above, you could stroll into that lion's den never having known about a lion, but it would still be dangerous! So awareness not only of what the emotion is, but why it's there, is vitally important. How much emphasis our perception places on that emotion depends on our experience with each situation. Courageous people are not absent of fear, they just persist despite it. Sometimes the most important thing we do is to choose a different behaviour, regardless of the emotions we are feeling. It's about knowing how much weight the fear, or whatever emotion is coming up, really deserves.

Resistance

In resistance, we label a feeling we are experiencing as undesirable. All emotions are created equally, and we know that in order to truly experience life we need all emotions – however, sometimes we have learned to not like particular feelings. When we resist emotions, or refuse to acknowledge them and the message they are carrying, we often block our flow in life.

Particularly common uncomfortable emotions include: fear, vulnerability, despair, sadness, anger, embarrassment, shame or guilt. By resisting these sometimes difficult feelings, we stop the wave of emotion. They get stuck, often in organs or cells, which is why an imbalance on the emotional level often shows up in the energetic or physical levels. This also connects to why people can get emotional releases when we open the energetic flow in the body, like in acupuncture or neural therapy. This doesn't mean that every emotion should be enjoyable, but if we just let our body experience it without any attachment or judgement to the emotion as good or bad, we can stay in much more balance and flow.

Why do we resist emotions? This is often a learned behaviour from a very young age. Maybe you were never taught to express a certain emotion and work through it. Or maybe certain emotions in your home were always shut down through "stop crying," or "stop fighting, just get along." The comfort or discomfort a parent has with a particular emotion is often learned from their childhood, unless the parent actively seeks to learn how to deal with and experience emotions more healthfully. They must learn how to be ok with their own emotions and how to appropriately express them.

A common resistance I see in my practice, and you may see in your life, is to anger. Some people may resist conflict because of their dislike of anger. Hence every time they feel this emotion or even see someone angry in front of them, they retreat, disengage and inevitably stop the flow of its expression – which may mean they may not deal with conflicts in their lives, or even worse, put up with behaviours that are hurtful or even harmful. Perhaps their parents also didn't like anger as they may have felt it ended up in physical pain, emotional pain or rejection, so they were never taught healthy ways to express anger.

In another circumstance, some of us can be quick to anger when our weak spots or insecurities are exposed, and then we project it on others: name calling, belittling or being abusive. This is a very unconscious way to handle anger – expressing the emotion, but in a way that is hurtful to others. This behavior means they are not being accountable and responsible for their own emotion. That person shifts the blame to someone else, rather than recognizing what the emotion is saying about them.

What might be more effective in dealing with anger? We first must recognize the anger, and maybe still even shout on our own, but not actually *at* anyone. Or we might viscously scribble on a piece of paper, or tense our body and then release, or scrunch a ball, or punch a pillow or boxing bag if need be, depending on our circumstances and the appropriateness of our outburst. It would be an interesting sight if every time a person felt a twinge of anger, they just randomly shouted it out: in the grocery store, at work or on an airplane. Although it might not be advisable, how comfortable other people would be with that expression, would say a lot about their own processes to express emotion. Of course this is largely cultural, but someone else should never be the brunt of our anger.

Knowing our internal reaction processes is equally important, in order to understand the root of the feeling – which goes beyond just the current situation, and rather looks at the reason… an injustice, a hurt, a misunderstanding. Dealing with those reasons then actually resolves the emotional context in the long term.

Whatever ways we choose to express our feelings – when we breathe through them and allow a release, we give our emotional knowledge the space to grow. You can then ask yourself:

1. Why did you get triggered?
2. What are the grooves of thought that led to that emotion?
3. Is there another emotion underneath your first reaction?
4. Maybe you were feeling defensive, because you felt your integrity was being attacked?
5. Maybe you were making assumptions about a circumstance?
6. Maybe you were taking someone else's response personally?

We are all responsible for our own emotions. No one can make you feel something, we have to own that all by ourselves.

Thus, the goal is to take your power back and become responsible for your own emotions. This is especially important if you feel like you are stuck in a situation or a cycle of destructive patterns. You may even use denial as your resultant coping mechanism to survive. You may have avoided the truth, stopped telling yourself the truth or simply made up a more suitable story to keep you in that pattern. Sometimes the most courageous thing you can do is get honest with yourself. The internal universal truth is always there, we're sometimes just afraid to ask. Afraid of what that feeling might mean for your life... try asking yourself, what are you tolerating in your life? For Robyn, it took reaching rock bottom before she started to make changes, but it doesn't have to go that far. It's just a choice you make – to look within and connect with how you are really feeling.

Robyn joined Alcoholics Anonymous® and Narcotics Anonymous® and started their 12 step process. She also asked for my help along the way to deal with the bigger issues physically, mentally and emotionally. Although it was hard, she really started to explore why she so badly needed to escape. Why she really couldn't even stand the idea of being vulnerable in relationships or be honest with herself. Through the process of 12 step, group counselling and one on one counselling, she had the courage to ask the hard questions – how did it come to this, and where was her responsibility and ownership of it all? What story had she been telling herself about her current reality? Where had she given her power away? How did she create that reality?

She was always an outgoing and determined person, now she finally used those attributes to step out into her life and get the things that she really wanted. She started an organic meal prep company from scratch, and took it to the point where she was able to leave her care aide job. In addition to counselling, she also started digging into books about codependency in order to understand why she choose to drink and do drugs in the first place. (I'd highly recommend "Codependency for Dummies" for more on that subject!) She started to find faith and explore her spiritual self.

Robyn started speaking in schools to young teens about the dangers and trials of a life of drugs and alcohol. Although her parents loved and supported her, they had a broken marriage which led to divorce, and it dramatically affected Robyn at an early age. The tension at home had left her feeling insecure and searching for affection in all the wrong places, so she had to heal from that experience as well. She then had to learn what it was like to have a healthy relationship. She started to learn to love herself – to be clean, not just for her daughter, but also for herself. We had many conversations about her need to be fully conscious of her behaviours and choices so that she could make different ones. She is still working on this each day – through self-reflection, counselling, reading books, meditation and practicing vulnerability, though with each step it gets easier and easier for her. She has transformed herself and how she lives her life. Her journey to wholeness has helped her become more aware of her behaviours, deal with vulnerability and its ensuing anxiety, grapple with being in a romantic relationship that doesn't allow for alcohol induced liquid courage, and most importantly, be the connected mother that she was always striving to be. She's now nearly four years clean, running a thriving and expanding business, and involved in a healthy loving long-term relationship.

Robyn is inspirational, just as anyone else can be too, if they choose to look more closely at the thoughts and emotions that are driving them to certain behaviours or patterns. To recognize what their thoughts and emotions are – constructs of their consciousness, not the essence of who they are. Who they are is much more important than what they do. We will see how this concept continues to apply to the next levels of health in the following chapters.

Emotions are there to help you understand a situation or thought, but they are just another piece in your health puzzle. They can lead you easily off course if you make every decision in your life from an emotional place. Think of what would happen if you only ever followed your emotions with every decision. It might be hard to hold down a job or stay in a relationship, as these are inevitability bound to let you down or disappoint you at one time or another. We may never be able to get to a goal or destiny if we always just follow what makes us feel good or comfortable. Emotions are necessary, and help with the momentum and perception of our lives. But they are also just another construct of our conscious experience of the now, just one part of our whole life experience.

THERAPIES FOR THE EMOTIONAL BODY:

1. Stress Management: There are countless books and techniques about managing stress. It is so important to reduce stress in order to initiate the parasympathetic nervous system and relaxation. We can never be in stress and relaxation simultaneously, so managing our stress and inducing down-time is essential. I have suggested all of these in my office: meditation, deep breathing, yin yoga, affirmations, counseling, guided imagery and support groups. Any of these methods can provide a way for the stress to be dealt with while still living amongst the stressors.

Some books to help with emotional healing that I often recommend, and patients love, include:
- *Don't Sweat the Small Stuff and It's All Small Stuff* by Richard Carlson
- *The Four Agreements* by Don Miguel Ruiz
- *The Gifts of Imperfection; Daring Greatly; Rising Strong* by Brené Brown
- *The Road Less Travelled* by Scott Peck, MD
- *The 5 Love Languages* by Gary Chapman
- *Declutter Your Mind* by Barrie Davenport and S.J. Scott
- *Untethered Soul* by Michael Singer
- *The Power of Now* by Eckhart Tolle
- *Keep Your Love On* by Danny Silk

---

2. Homeopathy: This treatment option also addresses the emotional level of healing. Homeopathy is a medicine that harnesses the energetic signature (the part that exists before matter) and helps to reveal to your body how it needs to heal. In classical homeopathy, specific remedies are found for a person by looking at their individual emotional and mental characteristics. The characteristics are cross referenced in order to create a treatment that is very unique to the person. The more mental and emotional symptoms that are used, rather than physical, the deeper the remedy will shift the person.

Classical homeopathy is an art, and it requires a very skilled homeopath to find a single correct remedy for an individual. It entails a detailed intake, often several hours in length, followed by ample time of repertorizing unique symptoms of the patient, before a remedy is chosen and prescribed. Classical homeopathy isn't used nearly as often today as things like homotoxicology, which uses combination remedies with similar principles but at lower potencies. These work more on the energetic and physical levels. Low dose remedies are also used for many physical ailments like headaches, hives or wound healing. In fact, in 1900, the United States had twenty-two Homeopathic medical schools, over 100 Homeopathic hospitals and more than 1,000 Homeopathic pharmacies. However, there has been a drastic and unfortunate decline in institutions across the board in North America in the last century due to the rise of pharmaceuticals. Homeopathy is still very popular and widely used in Europe and India.

3. Change our situation or perspective on stress: This is the only way to actually change our relationship to our stressors. While we could take some adrenal supplement for the rest of our lives, it would never touch why we are getting stressed. Making the needed changes are often the hardest things to do, but the most permanent and successful way to deal with stress. Sometimes we need change in our life, such as to our relationships or our workplace, in order to move into a place that is more in alignment with who we are, and is more supportive of our needs. However, I would challenge you to question whether this may just be a quick fix, and if the more deeply rooted stressor will follow you no matter the circumstances.

It's important to note that what makes you stressed is entirely different than what makes anyone else stressed. One person may worry about timelines or deadlines at work, another about personal interactions at work, and yet another about the type of work they are doing – the difference is their perspective, not the environment. When we challenge ourselves to look at the situation differently, then we can also instantly change how it affects us. Part of dealing with stress is realizing that no one can make you stressed, you own that all by yourself. To say that someone else does, is to give away all of your power. It's *your* body reacting, not someone else's, so it's *your* brain's interpretation of life, whether you are aware of it or not, that triggers the physiological stress response. We have the ability to change how we look at the world; to see events or situations as something that happens to us, or something that we create. Which feels more empowering and true? I'm not suggesting that bad things don't happen, even to good people, but I am suggesting that how we deal with it is entirely our own doing. See the list of books above for more resources to help you with shifting your perspective.

4. Choosing your words: Words have power, and the ones you use can be crippling or powerful. When moving into the space of being a conscious creator of your life, start owning your words. Which feels better? I have to go to work or I want to go to work? I should be gluten free or I choose to be gluten free? Use powerful words that instil courage, empowerment and a choice! When we use positive, motivating words (choose to, want to, or my needs are) instead of negative, dishonouring words (have to, should do, or obligated to) we feel more in control of our choices, ourselves and our lives. It's your life and your choice to own it. It can be that simple to change how we feel in our lives.

5. Emotional Language: Often we have a hard time identifying with their emotions because they literally don't have the vocabulary to

DR. ALANA BERG, ND

define it. Often, people list their top 5: happy, sad, angry, confused or scared. Yet, there is such a wide range of words to describe our feelings, and sometimes the very thing we need to do is just acknowledge it. Like a reactive toddler, when we are able to say, "I see you are disappointed that we weren't able to go to the park," they can quickly start to diffuse because their emotion has been acknowledged. In the case of a 2 year old, they haven't the maturity to have the language for their feelings, but how many adults do you know that act the same way?! It's a good practice to expand our emotional vocabulary so that we have the words to express how we feel.

Emotional Feeling Chart by Intensity

	Low	Medium	High
Happy	Content Peaceful Fine Mellow Glad Hopeful Confident	Good Cheerful Satisfied Proud Optimistic Joyful Open	Overjoyed Powerful Elated Excited Thrilled Ecstatic Delighted
Sad	Bored Indifferent Ignored Moody Sorry Lost Vulnerable Down	Upset Guilty Isolated Inferior Remorseful Distressed Empty Hurt	Disappointed Alone Hopeless Devastated Depressed Ashamed Despair Powerless
Angry	Uptight Irritated Touchy Distant Put out Sarcastic	Upset Mad Frustrated Resentful Jealous Skeptical	Infuriated Furious Hateful Outraged Seething Hostile
Afraid	Nervous Worried Unsure Timid Anxious Submissive Insecure	Frightened Threatened Shocked Embarrassed Rejected Overwhelmed Scared	Panicky Terrified Horrified Petrified Humiliated Worthless Fearful
Confused	Puzzled Undecided Uncomfortable Unsure	Disorientated Mixed up Disorganized Foggy	Dismayed Bewildered Desperate Trapped
Disgust	Disapproval Critical Judgmental Hesitant	Aversion Awful Avoidance Loathing	Revolted Detestable Revulsion Distain

Look at the chart provided, it can be a reference when you need more clarity, or a practice to challenge yourself to think of situations you can associate that feeling to. You may also find more charts online that you could download to your phone for a quick reference.

6. Counselling and psychotherapy: These therapies are effective for this layer of healing. They help you gain understanding and perspective about yourself. You don't know what you don't know, and talking with an unbiased professional can help you shed light on what is happening in your life. Bringing awareness of how you are responding to stress from the unconscious mind to the conscious mind is sometimes all that is needed to create healing. If you gain understanding into something about why you behave in certain ways – for example, your fear of rejection being a key to your inability to commit in a relationship – you may be able to transform this habit. By understanding that fear, you can see the emotion for what it is, and make a different choice in relationships. Other times, we may have to work harder to gain this insight. For example, in the case of using meditation to change thought patterns, most people need to make an extended, concerted effort in order to make it an effective practice.

There are many different styles and types of counselling and you should always make sure you find a style that is the right fit for you. Most importantly, your counsellor should be someone objective, that you can trust, who displays empathy and believes in your healing. They create a safe space to challenge you to gain insight into your life and teach you tools to become a more balanced, authentic you.

7. Desirable experience list: Lastly, in order to understand where we are going, we want to use our conscious mind to our benefit. There is a saying that if you're not dreaming, you're dying – which really means if we're not in a place of hope for what is yet to come, our souls are stuck and dying. Hope is a promise of things not yet seen. So it's a decision and an action to believe in your future.

What future? The one you are intentionally and consciously creating.

To do that, start by creating an *experiential* want list and/or vision board. I first heard about this concept from Vishen Lakhiani on Tom Bilyeu's Impact Theory program.[79] I agree with their statements that setting experiences is more important than specific goals. Goals can sometimes be too rigid and confined for the evolution of life. Rather, we want to attract and allow for the experience we desire. This also means that experience might not show up in the way we conceive. For example, I might say, "I want to have a million dollars!" Why? It's not actually about physically having a million dollars, but rather the experiences I am seeking that I believe a million dollars would create, such as freedom, abundance, ability to give at a great capacity, ability to focus on my purpose and passions, ability to travel. Those are experiences... but in the end I might not need a million dollars to get those experiences.

Or maybe you might say, "I want to own a sports car." Why? Because... "I want the feeling of driving fast, the feeling of being streamlined, or the ability to take my friends places in it."

Or another goal might be, "I want to be a mother or father." Why? Because..."I want to commit my life to someone other than myself and be invested in their development and care, or I want to leave a legacy, or I want to feel and give unconditional love."

Or maybe the goal is to have a healthy, disease-free body. Why? Because... "I can then fully participate in the life I want to live, challenge myself, be active or seek growth, rather than be clouded by pain or fatigue." This is an interesting concept; can you see the personal accountability behind the desire that the goal is asking for in this example? It's not about leaving it up to fate or chance, but recognizing the limitation that we already put on ourselves if we narrow the goal to something specific.

Examining the reasons for your desirable experiences can bring up a whole host of insecurities and fears, but it also shows what you must overcome. If you don't know why you want something, how can you "attract" it in your life – or in other words, how can God bring it to you?

I believe there is always a dynamic working together in the creation of your life – your actions, that demonstrate your intention to attract something you want or need – and God's action, those things that happen which life orchestrates but are outside of your direct influence. The purpose of asking yourself the question of *why*, is so that:

1. you understand where your desire comes from to have that something in your life,
2. you know which steps and actions are required for you to attract this, and finally
3. this understanding then allows you to be in a position of flow of intention so that opportunities can show up, or God can meet your desires, even if it doesn't end up looking exactly like you anticipated.

When you focus on the desired experience over the goal, this also removes the attachment and conditions you have to a specific outcome. Focusing on an outcome may actually lead to discouragement and a feeling of failure. Focusing on the desired experience leaves you open to opportunity and success, however it may show up. The experiences in life are all that we have in the end. Start to write those desires down or find pictures that represent them in a collage. Challenge yourself to get to 50… or 100!

As you can see, there are many methods for healing on the emotional level. In my own healing, I had to work through the story of perfectionism, stemmed in feelings of inadequacy. My deeply ingrained belief was that I needed to be perfect in order to be loved. This is when you are motivated to do things exceptionally well for *external reward* rather than *internal gratification*. The approval of others! It got me through medical school and gave me a work ethic like no other, but I was also incredibly hard on myself, especially if I perceived anything I did to be a failure. I grew up believing perfectionism was a requirement for success and acceptance. But all it brought me in my birthing experience was a sense of failure and shame. Thoughts like, "I've failed as a woman," "What will other people think," "I'm an inadequate mother," or "How can I be a good mother, when I resented and was traumatized by the birth my child," frequently ran through my mind. Although the traumatic birth experience was out of my control, my deeply ingrained belief that I needed approval from others required me to get it right, all the time – or I was sure I would face disgrace and shame! After much searching and processing, I finally understood that my mental dependency on perfection was causing the guilt feeling around my daughter's birth.

To heal from my trauma, stemming from this perfectionist belief, I also had to heal the relationship with my mom. You see, my mother is a perfectionist, due to her upbringing, which in turn was instilled in me. In my perception, I always thought I had to be perfect in order to be accepted and loved, and thus I always felt I couldn't let my parents down. When you are a perfectionist, you also tend to expect perfection from everyone around you (my poor husband)!

To heal, I had to be OK with letting my mom down and just being me, whether she really did or it was just my belief. At the end of the day it was "my story" – and deep down, I knew that she loved me no matter what. I had thrown in so many expectations into the relationship, that it often led me to disappointment. I had, therefore, to grieve the loss of this relational idea so that that I could create a new story of total acceptance and love. This was a painful truth and realization of how I needed to change. I understood that I just needed to be me.

Once I got through that grief, I was able to accept my mother for who she was, a beautiful loving human. I finally got to love her unconditionally (the very thing I thought I was searching from her). Only then could I let go and accept myself, flaws and all, and change my belief around perfection. Having two daughters of my own, this understanding has become particularly important to me. I know I never want them to grow up feeling that my love for them was conditional based on how well they did, or whether I agreed with their decisions.

This, of course, is a process for me, just like your healing is a process. But remember, you are the creator of your life. Would you rather do this intentionally or inadvertently? Either way, you are still creating it.

Summary

Our emotional body gives us context to our human experience in this world. Without emotions life would be flat and bland.

1. They are an important part of who we are, and they drive us forward in life with passion, excitement and motivation; therefore we do not want to avoid any of the messages our emotions are telling us.
2. However, it is important to understand that emotions are not truths, they are formed from our mental body, based on our past beliefs, experiences, and circumstances.
3. Hence, if we give too much emphasis to our emotions without realizing the limitations they may be creating, we can end up being steered off course.

We will discuss more in the next chapter, how these mental constructs, both conscious and unconscious, are the biggest determiners of our life experience. In understanding the deeper level of healing, you will really start to harness the power and ability to transform your life. You can be the conscious and courageous creator of your own life story.

TEN

Fourth Level: Mental Body

"Be careful how you think; your life is shaped by your thoughts."
~Proverbs 23:4

When Carrie brought Lucas in to see me, he was having numerous stomach concerns. He often vomited after meals and repeatedly complained of stomach pains. When we dug deeper, I realized he had actually had issues since he was an infant. His mother recounted how he had projectile vomiting starting within the first few months of introducing formula. She noticed early on that dairy made him very ill, so she removed it completely from his diet by the age of two. He continued to struggle though, and had a hard time swallowing anything that was large without feeling like it was getting stuck. At the age of nine, everything he ate still had to be in tiny little pieces. I believed the difficulty swallowing was likely due to some inflammation, scar tissue or damage in the esophagus, possibly even eosinophilic esophagitis. Without a scope at that point, we couldn't know for sure, so we started with food testing, where several food sensitivities came up, including gluten, soy, peanut, corn and of course, dairy. I also began some digestive healers to help to improve his stomach symptoms.

During this course, however, I sensed there was some deeper healing that needed to occur, since the symptoms started at a very young age. His mother did report a fairly stressful pregnancy. We did a Bodytalk session, and in that appointment, what came up was an unconscious feeling of deep sadness from a loss of connection between mother and son when she stopped breastfeeding at three weeks of age and turned to formula to supplement. She didn't feel she was producing enough milk, nor did she feel supported emotionally with the difficulty nursing. She felt remorseful and internally conflicted about not continuing to nurse. It was shortly after that he started becoming colicky and projectile vomiting, and she responded by primarily avoiding dairy because of his extreme reactions.

The fourth level of healing resides in the Mental Body – the mind that gives awareness of one's own existence through the collection of thoughts, feelings, sensations and perceptions.

In the analogy of the horse drawn carriage from earlier, we talked about the driver being your director... by directing your thoughts. It gives you the required mental awareness to navigate and move forward in life, to be able to make choices and decisions, to figure out problems and avoid danger. We need the mind. The mind is so miraculous at its work, that much of the time we don't even need to be focusing on our tasks and yet we still perform them. This means most of what we do comes from the subconscious mental mind. For example, once you've learned to walk, or ride a bicycle or learn any new skill, you don't have to relearn this task every time you try it. Imagine telling your leg which muscles to fire and how to take a step each and every time you walk?! Our brain needs to keep space free for new information; otherwise we'd be mentally exhausted with even the slightest task. Hence our regular habits and perceptions are controlled by the subconscious mind.

Many of us get caught up in thinking we are our minds. That we are our thoughts, and the mind controls us. I have had many patients over the years say that they "just can't turn off their brain." It keeps them up at night, it makes them anxious and they have a hard time resting because their mind is always going.

The mind can be divided into three layers: the conscious, subconscious and unconscious. This concept was developed extensively by the famous psychologist Sigmund Freud. It is a simple, yet accurate and concise method of understanding how the mind works.

1. _Conscious mind_: This is the part of the mind that we can access. It is mostly the accumulation of our streams of thought. It is simply a part of our awareness, the one we can direct and control. Awareness of what is going on in your surroundings, your body, your mind and your heart.

This is the level of the mind that many of us refer to as self. We can only access what we are aware of, so logically it means these are things we can talk about and know. We can only know what we can access.

The conscious mind is where we have reactions, rational thought, willpower, critical thinking and long term memory. It is where our intellect resides. The intellect observes a situation, interprets it, and then understands it so we can create a response or a decision.

The conscious mind is connected to our Ego, which in psychology is really referring to "I" or "me." Ego is the collection of definitions or labels we apply to ourselves. It is our self-described identity. Ego is formulated from our personal experiences and beliefs about our personalities, abilities and talents. From a historical standpoint, ego has been thought of as being required to control impulses and desires, but it is also always looking for self-preservation and protection. Its goal is to survive – which means it is also very self-focused. This may not always be in our best interests in the long term for growth, relationships or deeper understanding! Imagine if our main motivation was always to protect ourselves from being hurt – from fears, rejection, abandonment, judgment, embarrassment, guilt or shame? Or if in every decision we made, we only had ourselves in mind? Ego would keep us in a very self-serving, limited, never changing box if it had the chance.

The mind is excellent at being able to analyze, rationalize and create logic where needed, which is why it is necessary for life. But if we understand the motives of the mind, particularly the ego, and recognize that we can, in fact, control it, then we can be free from its endless chatter – that nagging voice that always wants to throw its two cents in on any subject.

Our conscious mind, although very active, comprises about 10% of the mental body. The majority of our mind's capacity resides in the subconscious and unconscious mind. The conscious mind is just the tip of the iceberg.

2. *Subconscious mind*: This level of the mind is the part where habitual patterns and responses lie, just below the surface of our awareness. However, the subconscious is also a part of our awareness, as we can access it if we try – but other than the occasional glimpse, it is ultimately not under our conscious control.

The subconscious is connected to your short term memory. It runs the active memories you're currently using – like how to walk, talk, ride a bike or drive a car. One of the subconscious' most important jobs is to act as the interface between the conscious and unconscious mind. This relationship can be described as follows: "The unconscious constantly communicates with the conscious mind via our subconscious, and is what provides us with the meaning to all our interactions with the world, as filtered through your beliefs and habits. It communicates through feelings, emotions, imagination, sensations, and dreams."[80] Thus, the subconscious acts as a filter for the external world: interpreting senses, and influencing behaviors, feeling and habits.

3. *Unconscious mind*: The unconscious mind is the vast part of the mind that we cannot access directly through conscious aware thought, but it dictates how we *frame* our thoughts and feelings. It consists of our preconceived belief systems, life experiences and stored memories. Without these, we could not create context for what is in front of us. This is why we all see and feel things differently; our experiences and beliefs are different.

The unconscious mind is merely a tape recorder of our life experiences and perceptions, but it is not the essence of us. It shapes our perspective in how we frame the world, but it is not a dynamic being. We don't think about how we respond to conflict, for example, we just react. That reaction is based on what we've seen in previous conflicts, how we were taught to deal with conflicts, and what the outcomes of our previous behavioural choices in conflict.

We may not even like what we have on that recorder – how we react or the habits we have – but no matter how much you yell at it, it doesn't respond. It's not until you press re-record that the unconscious dialogue can change.

How is the unconscious mind formed?

Many of these unconscious definitions of our reality come from our childhood, when we were just learning how to figure out the world around us. For example, every child has a great need to feel safe and loved. As children, this is largely a situation that they cannot provide for themselves, especially at a young age. But what happens if that security is shaken – maybe a mother or father was either physically or emotionally absent, maybe the child was not able to bond to an adult in early childhood due to abandonment, adoption or neglect, or perhaps there was a natural disaster where consistency was not available. The child's basic initial ability to trust another human being and in turn, show love and be loved would have been compromised. How might that shape their perspective later on in life? Maybe they would have troubles trusting others, showing their emotions, setting boundaries or asking for what they need? These problems could cause broken relationships, crippling anxiety, passive or aggressive behaviours (depending on their demeanour), or perhaps a constant need to control and manipulate their surroundings. There are many examples such as these that demonstrate how unconscious patterns can develop.

However, this doesn't mean that you are a product of your childhood – rather, the unconscious mind just provides an understanding of *why* you do what you do. The unconscious mind is the motivator for all your behaviours; personal, internal, and instinctual desires.

Learning about your belief systems isn't about laying blame on someone else, like your parents or caregivers. Your parents were no different in how they formed their patterns and beliefs. You'd have to credit them for everything good about you, as well as blame them for everything bad, if we were to only look at our unconscious self as a product of our upbringing. It's not about creating an excuse for undesirable behaviour, but rather just fostering our understanding. In the end, whether we choose to be aware of our motives or not, we are still ultimately the ones responsible for our actions.

Everyone is at a different level of consciousness or awareness. The more aware we become of ourselves by asking questions about our own actions, the more responsible we will become for our own behaviour. All too often, people live their lives completely unaware of why they do what they do, or say what they say. They may think that's just the way the world works, and they are helpless to change it, even if they don't like it. That statement I hope you are beginning to understand is highly inaccurate!

When the world seems heavy and hurtful and traumatic, it might first of all help to try to look at the world a little differently. If you are able to understand that every human being is inherently doing the best job he or she can, with what they know and understand, then you can start to feel compassion for everyone. Now I didn't say that they are doing the best that *you* can, but rather the best that *they* can. Brené Brown discusses this wonderfully in her book, *Rising Strong*.[81]

So often, our judgement of others is based on our perceived ability that we could "do better." Yet, we are not them, so how do we know? Life experiences, personal circumstances, coping mechanisms, support systems and personalities all dictate how that person responds to the world around them. Every single person's unconscious self is different from everyone else's. We are all unique. Ever hear that saying, it's easy to judge until you walk a mile in someone else's shoes? So even what you might perceive would be your worst behavior in their circumstance, might actually be their best that they are able to do at that moment in time, for whatever reason. They may even know better, but because of *their* own stories and limiting beliefs, this is the choice they feel they must make.

Since the 1950s, studies have been performed that look at criminal activity and the perpetrator's justification. *Why did they do it?* There is what has been described as the neutralization theory, which has evolved over the last sixty years. This essentially identifies the offender's common justifications for the criminal activity they have committed – whether that is murder, rape, robbery or any other offense. This theory explains how the felons too have a story – maybe they feel their behavior was accidental, not their intention, motivated by forces beyond their control – or they were a victim of their circumstances, a product of their environment, the crime was deserved by the victim and so on.[82] Anyone could have a story of justification for why they don't have to be accountable for themselves, and that anything could be permissible. This might be an extreme example, but I want you to understand the universal principle: we all have a "reason" for why we do what we do.

When we really grapple with that realization, we can actually look at a person that hurt us with compassion. How broken does that person have to feel to hurt another person? This is an axiom, or universal truth – all we really want as human beings is to be loved, feel connected, be accepted and be truly known. Even the people that have hurt you have that exact same desire in their soul. Perhaps it's just been distorted in some way, and the only way they can change is if they too choose to change. We cannot force others to change, become personally aware, or become responsible for themselves. Likewise, if you wish to change, you must desire it. No one is going to fix your unconscious limiting beliefs, you are solely responsible for desiring that change and making it happen.

So, since it is our personal responsibility to understand those internal drives, do we say "That's just the way I am, and I can't change it," or do we say "Hey, maybe this isn't the most skilful way of doing things." Maybe it's time to move away from our childhood perspectives, whose main desire was to satisfy our basic needs: food, clothing, shelter, safety, security, acceptance, belonging and love. We need to recognize that how our needs were met was based on our childhood environment, and whatever adaptive way seemed to satisfy those basic needs the best.

In Lucas's case, he was much too young to have any conscious awareness of the circumstances of his mom's pregnancy, and her struggles with nursing him. Yet unconsciously, the memory of a disconnection from his mother remained.

In the Bodytalk session with Lucas, we made an interesting discovery – the dairy reaction was manifesting an unconsciously stored feeling of grief due to the torn emotional bond with his mom. Milk represented the bond. I took him through the procedure of clearing this association and synchronizing the body – essentially helping the body to reprogram a new truth. I said that we should give it a couple weeks and then retest for dairy. She did, and surprisingly dairy didn't show up as a food sensitivity. She slowly and cautiously reintroduced dairy with him. Again, to their surprise, no reaction. A child that would normally have instant stomach pain and vomiting from dairy, had no reaction! She continued to allow little bits of dairy here and there and still no reactions. He still couldn't eat gluten, soy and peanuts, but the dairy was ok! Now, some four years later, after a scope completion which did reveal a stricture, he can still eat dairy, and has never had a reaction to it again. We are continuing to support proper digestion and esophageal healing, as there is now residual damage from the reflux history. This is an example of how healing the body on an unconscious level can bring about physical results. This is one of the deepest levels of healing you can tap into.

Changing the Unconscious Mind:

As adults, shifting the unconscious mind will affect every behaviour, thought, feeling, sensation and response that is essential for our wellness and growth. Actually, I believe the key **to becoming a mature adult is to stop living completely unconsciously, and start becoming aware** of your own behaviours, and how they are framing your current reality. These unconscious thoughts construct all labels or judgments of the world around you and within you. When you really become aware, regardless of the cards you were dealt, you learn to communicate effectively and express your desires and needs without the "stories" behind them. You can use your conscious mind as an advantage, perpetuating the beliefs and stories you want to create.

How we judge our current circumstances can come from favourable memories, that might give us a more positive or optimistic view, or from more uncomfortable ones, that might slant our view to be more closed, jaded or pessimistic. It's not the environment that determines our reality, but rather how we look at it.

1. How are we filling in the blanks?
2. What are we labeling?
3. What judgements are we making about others and ourselves?
4. How many of us actually ask ourselves, why we do what we do?

We *are* answering these questions *unconsciously* over and over again in every single reaction and interaction we have, we just aren't aware of it. These beliefs colour our perspective. How we interpret our reality is ultimately our own responsibility!

We can all have all sorts of negative self-talk inside of us. Sometimes this happens without us even realizing it. We might say, "This always happens to me, I don't even know why I try." Or maybe we say, "I knew this eventually would happen," or "It had to be too good to be true," or "I'm not lovable, of course this would happen." In these scenarios, at some level we're waiting for the other shoe to drop because we're anticipating some sort of failure to happen, perhaps because of a previous experience. Thus, rather than seeing the moment as the present without judgement, we expect it to follow a pattern from the past. Hence, we are unconsciously bringing our past forward. Like the situation when someone self-sabotages a relationship because they just know at some point that other person will leave – they are convinced, based on past experiences that they're destined to be alone.

Anticipating our future based on past beliefs can be particularly destructive. Subliminally we are looking for reinforcement of our old belief systems, so that our ego can stay intact and in control. The ego, remember, is the part of our conscious mind that is all about survival and self-preservation. It would be a big blow to our ego if we accepted the responsibility for how our life is playing out right now... phew, it will want to avoid that at all costs! It's much easier to avoid, evade and blame.

Healing Trauma:

In chapter six, I mentioned that trauma often affects our health on the mental level. Trauma may happen in an instant – from an accident, injury, disaster or violence – or over time,-from a troubling relationship, abuse, illness or stress. The trauma from this event or experience is stored in our core memory banks. The memory then affects each and every level: physical, energetic, emotional, mental and even the spiritual. The deeper the health imbalance, the more levels will correspondingly be affected. If we're not actively focused on trying to heal trauma and its related pain, it can cause a more permanent unconscious wound, that seeps and stings throughout our lives, and colours every experience we have. When we are ready to deal with this pain, it is merely a choice – if we are suffering mentally, emotionally or physically, how long does it take before we decide we have had enough? For me, the physical and emotional trauma of my daughter's birth went on to colour my perspective on being a mother. Neglecting to take the required time to heal ended up affecting all aspects of my body: my energy, my vitality, my brain and my nerves. It took me to experience physical symptoms before I recognized my need for healing, but it didn't have to get to that point.

Now I want you to understand fully, that we don't need to carry the trauma forward. It is a part of our past, but those wounds do not need to define us. As humans, we all have hurts, but when we can't move past them, we often continue to hurt ourselves and others. As Carolyn Myss talks about in *Why People Don't Heal, And How They Can*, when we carry these wounds we stop our ability to heal.[83] Sometimes we even wear the wound like a badge to keep the world at arm's length, allowing us to not be accountable for our own lives. To unconsciously use these wounds as an excuse to stay where we are and behave as we do, become a justification.

It's amazing the behaviors a person may perform when feeling justified or even deserving – such as in the criminal studies we discussed above. How do you think good people, who we inherently all are, come to behave badly? They have chosen to justify a falsehood, a story that has distorted the truth. In turn, they feel it is their right to perform actions that may even be unspeakable. As humans, we have all been hurt, we have all felt pain. That's what makes us the same, not different. It's what we then do with the pain – use it as fuel for growth or for destruction? Sometimes, trauma and pain can be hidden gifts to help us on our path of discovering who we are really meant to be.

The most inspirational and moving stories that encourage us to grow in positive ways include stories of heroism, bravery and courage. These people overcome, persevere, and succeed not because of their adversity, but despite it. Gandhi, The Dalai Lama, Nelson Mandela, Jesus Christ, Oprah Winfrey, Albert Einstein, Thomas Edison, Vincent Van Gogh, Franklin Roosevelt, Ludwig van Beethoven: these are inspirational, impactful people, who are human, no different than you and I. They just chose to not let the pain, suffering or adversity they felt define their futures. It's not what you've been through that defines you, but rather how you've overcome them. The option to be your best self in this world is not because the world owes it to you, but rather because you owe it to the world. What gifts, talents and abilities are in you to give?

The key to shifting the pain of trauma is forgiveness of others and often of self. Grace is the knowledge that we can be forgiven – that we all make mistakes and trip up. Grace is the greatest gift from God. Forgiveness can be a hard pill to swallow, but understand that this concept is not about saying that what happened was ok – it is not approval or even acceptance of what has happened. It isn't about needing to like or reconnect to that person that has wronged you. It is about you recognizing that you are choosing not to continue to carry the hurt or pain or fear or anger or resentment anymore. Holding on to it only hurts you.

When I moved through my personal traumatic labour experience, I begrudgingly realized I had to forgive myself: for not knowing every-thing, for being imperfect, for not being prepared, for pushing myself, and for being vulnerable like everyone else. I also had to forgive the midwife that didn't give me the tools and information I thought I needed. I had to forgive the Obstetrician who I felt didn't treat me humanely in my delivery experience. These shortcomings were all based on my own perspective, of course, not necessarily on actual truth, but I needed to let them go in order to be free from the pain emotionally and allow for my body to heal physically. I needed to heal, and it wasn't about anyone else. We all did the best job we could, under those circumstances. Forgiveness was a choice I made in order to move forward with my life without fear, resentment, and shame. Our bodies are designed to heal; we just have to remove the obstacles, so we can find our cure.

THERAPIES FOR THE CONSCIOUS MIND:

"The Soul always knows what to do to heal itself. The challenge is to silence the mind."
~Caroline Myss

1. Controlling the mind:

a. Firstly, it's important to understand that by control I don't mean stopping any incessant thought – we are human and thinking is part of the deal. Rather, it's about recognizing what those thoughts are, then consciously and intentionally choosing whether or not you are going to pursue them. You probably will know whether or not to follow the thought by how it makes you feel: anxious, sad, angry, lonely, guilty or fearful? Mental consciousness is tied closely to the emotional body, because the mind's perception of the environment creates the emotions we feel, which helps us interpret our environment. The thoughts are a construct of your consciousness, designed to get your attention and give information – how much power you give them is, believe it or not, up to you.

b. The second concept in controlling your mind is to examine why you are having these thoughts, especially if they are occurring continually? Are there some unresolved hurts that haven't been attended to? Are there some underlying fears that need to be addressed? Is there a message the body is trying to convey? Consciousness isn't an absence of thoughts, but rather an awareness of them, and then choosing what path to follow. We spend a lot of time thinking about ways to control our environment so that we ultimately can feel better or more comfortable, when in reality we can't control a lot of what's going on around us. The only thing that we can control is our mind!

c. Meditation is the technique that works at showing you how you can control your mind. There are several different types of meditation. Some include:

i. Zen meditation: This technique trains you to focus your mind on something specific: your breath, a sensation in the body, an emotion or a sound. The goal is to actually create an absence of thoughts, no mind chatter whatsoever. But this takes a great concerted effort, so would be very difficult to perform and still go on with your day simultaneously. There is a reason that when people meditate or pray, they are doing nothing else, no movement, eyes closed, no distractions. When a person learns to meditate, only then can they fully understand that you can actually exist in a thought free state... that you are not your thoughts! Wow, so freeing.

ii. Visualization meditation: This involves a guided meditation or visualization with a particular goal – like healing, stress release or sleep. This can be a very good meditation for beginners as you are focused on listening to someone else guiding the practice.

iii. Mindfulness meditation: This involves observing your current awareness and the present moment, noticing when thoughts arise. Then without judgment, returning to the meditation practice.

iv. Mantra meditation: This is a traditional practice in which you repeat out loud or silently a mantra like "Om" to bring you into a state of peace and calm.

v. Movement meditation: This method involves rhythmical movement like yoga and Qi Gong, or even walking, playing music or gardening, that creates an inner calm and connection to the now. You may relate to this when people talk about being in "the zone". This concept refers to being so intently focused on a game, sport or other activity that you become fully immersed in it – time doesn't seem to exist outside of the activity. You are in the flow. It can also be when you are doing something you are deeply excited and passionate about. You lose yourself in the moment, and forget to think, you just do, fully present in that instant. But as soon as you think, "Hey wait, where's my thoughts?", guess what, they're there again, ready to take you out of your moment and into some other space and time.

The mind is so often in another dimension, either dwelling on the past, or planning for the future, but the present is actually where the peace is. It's in this moment, when we are connected to our present moment, that helps us put our lives and our "stories" in perspective.

2. Determine your story: An effective way to work through your incessant thoughts or emotions is to examine their corresponding belief systems a little. First you want to write down the story you are telling yourself, no holds barred. As the brilliant author and researcher Brené Brown talks about in her books about vulnerability, like *Rising Strong*, she calls it your "shitty first draft or SFD"[84]. We want to get down the story of what has wounded you, or is keeping you stuck in the pattern that you have recognized that you want to change – whether that is a fear, an unhealthy behaviour, a crippling memory or anything else. From there we want to work to understand its roots. Here are some questions to work through to create a greater understanding after you've written out your "story". Eventually you will be able to answer them in your head when this becomes a practice.

- How does this story make me feel? Shameful, unworthy, fearful, alone?
- What assumptions am I making? Do I think I know what other people are thinking or doing?
- What am I taking personally? Am I internalizing someone else's story or even a cultural perspective that is untrue?
- What am I projecting? What am I putting out there that contributes to this story?
- What are my beliefs around this? Do I feel like I don't deserve to be happy, that I'm destined to be alone, that I will never be good enough, that people won't really accept me if they know me?
- How am I creating this? What behaviours and attitudes are perpetuating this "reality"?
- What is the underlying element of truth? Do I just want to be accepted, loved or understood?
- Is there something I need to let go of or someone I need to forgive?
- What narrative do I want to create? If I could, how would I change this story?
- What am I ready to change to create this? And how? What

actions can I make right now?

3. Day map: Another activity to utilize your conscious mind to work towards your desired outcome is to map out your perfect day so that you have an idea of what circumstances you're trying to create in your life. If you had the ability to completely set up your average day, what would it look like? Would you be working the same job? What time would you get up and go to bed? What type of foods would you be eating? What sort of things would you be doing? Would you be by yourself or with other people? Many of us plan big end goals but very few day to day goals, and what they would look like. How would your end goal make a difference to your daily life? Believe it or not, this activity can be much harder than it seems. The more detail you put down the better – remember, you are consciously creating your life.

THERAPIES FOR THE UNCONSCIOUS MIND:

The more we become aware of our unconscious selves, the more transformation we can create in our lives. There are several modalities of healing we can access to assist us.

Our intuition is believed to be connected to the unconscious mind, through the subconscious mind. It is the process of perceiving or knowing something without your conscious reasoning of it, an internal knowing that is not from a conscious area of our mind or a rational concept of self. This intuitive knowing is also likely affected by the body's perceptions, called the psychophysiology of the body, like of the heart, creating messages to the unconscious mind.[85] This is researched extensively by the Heart-Math Institute, in order to explain intuition by heart-mind messaging.[86] Either way our body creates an intuitive knowing, and as such accessing intuition is an essential piece to understanding the realms of the unconscious. Have you ever had the feeling someone is staring at you from across the room? This is not from a thought, nor a feeling, it's a sense. The unconscious plane is absent of thought, hence it's more of a knowing, that gut feeling. Finding a meditative state, like in the example of mindful meditation, may also access the unconscious self. When we quiet the mind chatter and allow a space for the knowing within to reveal itself, we are accessing our intuition: through an image, a colour, a feeling, a thought, a sense... anything.

There is a really great book called *The Untethered Soul* that helps you work through the prospect of understanding and controlling the inner workings of your mind, so that you can find that "mind-less" state. It teaches you to be able to reveal understanding from the unconscious self, all the reasons why you do what you do. We need to be in a state of self-awareness in order to reveal unconscious thoughts, ideas or beliefs, to make sense of the nonsensical. When you start to have that awareness, you start to see the purpose and alignment of all things around you. You are here on a journey of growth and self-discovery, and everything going on around you is to your benefit on that journey. The unconscious thoughts are like mirrors and stories that are playing out to get you to see something or reveal a message. What will they reveal? Maybe the answer to the bigger questions in your life – not accessible from our rational, logical mind. That mind is full of thoughts and their corresponding emotional pulls. Rather, those intuitive answers will come from the unconscious mind, which is the greater influence in our everyday life.[87]

There is no such thing as coincidence. Things don't always happen for a reason that we can understand, but they do happen for a purpose. There is significance in all things. Each event and situation is moving you towards your greater purpose. I can't tell you how many times I've "randomly" and casually met someone in my life, who later ended up becoming hugely connected to my life. At the time, I had no real understanding of the significance of the meeting, but I often had a sense that it was a meaningful connection. And in due time, as the situation unfolded, it revealed a deeper connection. I sometimes sit in awe at how life comes together!

1) Hypnotherapy: This technique has been around for centuries. It is used to put a person into a deeply relaxed state where the conscious mind is no longer in charge, in order to gain access directly to the subconscious mind, which in turn is threaded to the unconscious. Imagine the unconscious mind as a tape recorder, just storing all of our beliefs, stories and experiences. We cannot get that tape recorder to stop playing the old tune we've recorded on it by yelling at it and saying, "Stop that! I don't want to hear that song again!" The song that plays all those old negative thoughts, worries or fears. Rather, we need to re-record it. Hypnotherapy works much like that. Recording a new, more desirable belief system through the power of suggestion while you are in a hypnotic state. Of course, the new "song" will not stick if we continue to repeat the same experiences over and over, without shifting our overall perspective, but it can work well to start the process of change. This method has been highly successful for weight loss, smoking cessation and other addictions.

2) Family constellations: This work is based on Bert Hellinger's methodology. It is derived from the basic understanding that every human being wants to feel loved and belong. Therefore, conflicts and traumas in a family can create generational issues because of that basic need not being met. When there has been a significant event – such as a death, murder, betrayal, trauma, abuse, abortion, miscarriage, serious illness – there can be a rift in a family dynamic. Thus there may need to be some generational healing. It is believed that until this is resolved in the particular family, the circumstances may even repeat throughout the generations to come. The goal of this therapy is to identify what conflict is unresolved in a family unit, then dynamically create a space of healing. This is done through using guided role play to resolve the event for all the family members. Remember that on the unconscious plane, time is irrelevant. So healing can happen now, even if the event is long past. I have both led and witnessed this therapy first hand and can say that it is quite remarkable how people are affected by it and are able to finally find a release for the traumatic event or conflict.

3) Timeline therapies: We can never change what has happened to us, only how we now feel about it. In this method, shown to me by author and educator Josep Soler, patients are first helped to access a particular unconscious initial event or trigger. This event is continually triggering a response in the present reality by drawing the past forward, so the goal of the therapy is to provide a state of release. Even if you don't consciously know what root event is needing to be addressed, the body, in its infinite wisdom, does. Through various questions, techniques and invoked muscle responses, we can bring that conflict forward. The healing then comes from having a more conscious perception of the event's effects in the present. Healing also comes from the freedom of forgiveness. While timeline therapy can be done in a number of ways, the overall process is remarkable for fostering a release that patients can immediately feel. Specifically, the healing is successful in dealing with deep ingrained emotions like anxiety, rejection or shame that perhaps have unknown origins.

4) Bodytalk®: This method was developed by Dr. John Valtheim, DC, and taps into the body's agenda of healing through muscle testing techniques. The practitioner is simply asking yes or no questions to the body and uses the determined muscle response to identify the answer, in order to be able to understand the agenda of the body. Hence, through this systematic method, the practitioner accesses unconscious dynamics that need to be integrated and balanced for the body to regain function on many levels of healing. This is a very peaceful and passive process for the patient, but is also enlightening, as it shows what the body is actually processing and clearing.

5) Psychokinesiology: In this therapy created by Dr. Dietrich Klinghardt, we are attempting to reveal emotional, unconscious imprints that we have stored in our bodies, which are typically associated with a particular organ. These imprints can be caused by experiences we've had, projections of others' emotions towards us, or by being a close witness to an event that didn't directly happen to us, but we were affected by. This comes up a lot in family dynamics. Here are a few examples:

- You take on a feeling of resentment that your parent actually felt, due to a disappointing event they experienced in their life.
- Someone's anger was projected onto you and you unconsciously accepted it and started to manifest that anger yourself.
- You experienced a traumatic event in your own life with a strong negative emotion, like guilt or shame for example, and the event and its associated emotions got locked into your belief system.

In psychokinesiology, the practitioner finds the key conflict via biofeedback, then supports the patient in giving the body permission to let it go. This therapy allows the body to orient itself back to its initial state of wholeness, regaining function both energetically and physically. Many of us unknowingly carry many different imprints.

6) Theta Healing®: In this therapy developed by Vianna Stibal, the practitioner is looking to achieve a theta brain wave state (dream state) in order to get a sense of the patient's individual potential healing process. The practitioner taps into this awareness, and then achieves an understanding of the purpose of the illness or imbalance. They can then declare a way for the system to find healing.

7) Tapping therapies: Emotional Freedom Technique is probably one of the most common tapping therapies. It was created by Gary Craig, and involves tapping a series of ten Chinese meridian points while the patient focuses on a specific problem. Afterwards, the patient rates the intensity of the problem, and the procedure is repeated until the intensity is reduced. Patients can even be taught to do this on their own to help them deal with negative or unwanted symptoms, thoughts or emotions. This method has been successfully used for chronic pain, anxiety, fears and phobias, addictions, trauma, depression and many more conditions.

8) Somatic healing: This is a field of talk therapy that was created by Dr. Peter Levine. It attempts to bridge the gap between the body and the unconscious mind. It works to relieve the symptoms of trauma-related health problems, including PTSD, by focusing on the patient's perceived body sensations. The premise is that these traumas are being held or locked in by the physical body as a somatic (material) experience. The goal is to release the trapped survival energy in the body to restore health and balance.

9) Heart Math®: An infrared sensor is used to measure your heart rate variability, in order to understand your physical, mental and emotional resilience. Equalized breathing is then performed with the purpose of balancing your sympathetic and parasympathetic nervous systems. This in turn allows for an awareness of your heart with the goal of achieving a state of coherence. Coherence does two things: first it allows for the bringing forth of emotions that are held inside, and secondly there is exchange of information from the heart and mind. Through this, the end result is being able to intuitively access the unconscious mind and the perceptions of the body into your consciousness. This offers you more clarity and allows you access to healing from within. This therapy is used extensively in conditions associated with the nervous system: such as stress, ADHD (attention deficit or hyperactive disorder), PTSD (post-traumatic stress disorder), chronic pain, hypertension, and many mental health conditions from depression, anxiety, to OCD (obsessive compulsive disorder).

10) Shamanic Journeying: Traditional shamanic journeys are performed whereby the practitioner or shaman is attempting to restore power back to the person. They typically enter into a deep relaxation state or trance, assisted by drumming or other techniques, where they will receive healing visions and guidance with the support of their spirit animals. This is a traditional practice amongst many Native American cultures, though variations are practiced globally.

There are many other methods not mentioned in this book, that also access the unconscious level to bring about awareness and healing. What is common amongst many of these therapies is the utilization of the practitioner's intuition to gain understanding. Intuition, as we discussed previously, is what some call the sixth sense. Intuition is not something that only a select few have, we all have it. Some may have it more developed and nurtured than others, but we are all capable of being intuitive. Children are probably the most prime examples of intuitive human beings, as they are often hyper aware and receptive to their environments, way beyond their years and understanding. However, modern society's emphasis on "rational logical thought" has often dictated that we override this sense. Hence, many people feel disconnected from their innate awareness. Do not lose hope, it can be developed.

We simply must start to learn to trust our intuition – that sense of knowing what we need and what is right for us – not because someone tells us so, but it feels right in our gut. Most importantly, as you are reading though this chapter, your intuition will be telling you if you need healing in this area. Consider the following:

1) Is this chapter speaking to you? In either a good or even bad way?
2) If so, there may be some healing required here. Choose a modality that *resonates* with you (aka instinctively gets your attention) and a practitioner to help you.
3) Ensure you trust this practitioner and their intentions. Are they true? As someone who works in the healing arts, I can tell you that having a confident, grounded practitioner as a source of support, is critically important in the healing process. They should have a pure and loving intent, even though you are paying for services.
4) It is also important to ensure that you are spiritually aligned, in faith or even religion, with your practitioner in order to be open and be receptive to someone speaking into your life on this level. You need to be able to trust how they practice and the corresponding healing that occurs.

Summary

As discussed earlier, the conscious mind is how we perceive and understand the world around us. This is shaped by our past experiences, belief systems, attitudes and assumptions. It is also highly influenced by the unconscious self (the things we are not aware of) and filtered through the subconscious. The unconscious shapes our personal reality of how we understand the world to be. As such, each of our experiences, attitudes and belief systems are unique to ourselves – therefore, so is each existence. So when people say, "This is my truth," what they are really saying is "This is my reality in the way that I see it".

It would make sense that if we each have our own truths, then we might want to change our reality if those truths are not serving us. For example, you might say, "My truth is that I have cancer and my parents had cancer, therefore I knew this would be my lot in life. I know this to be my reality and eventually it was going to happen". Does that belief system serve you?

Or perhaps you might say, "My mom was always worrying and anxious when I was young, and it made for a very unstable, edgy childhood. I can't help that I also deal with mental health issues. I worry about everything, and the truth is I will always have anxiety; I have to just learn to manage it since I can't stop it." Is that the reality you want to continue to live?

What if I told you that you don't have to? Remember, everyone's reality is different, so there is a possibility to change yours too. Whatever you believe becomes your way of life. One person may say, "I have to work hard and sacrifice to be remotely successful," and another may say, "Success is about flow and freedom and abundance, and I deserve that." There may be little difference between these two people other than what they believe to be true, but their experience of life would feel quite different..

There are many therapies out there meant to access our mental level of healing. How do you know which one may be right for you? Chances are that if you participate in any one of these methods, the details that come up will be new to you, as they will come from the unconscious. You will experience a greater knowing that helps you make more sense of your life, without completely understanding why, or even how to fully articulate what has happened. It's like someone telling you something for the first time, but somehow, you already knew. Even talking about the unconscious can be very hard because it's not about our logical, rational brain.

For the purposes of this book, I am only scratching the surface of all that can be known and understood about the complexities of our unconscious nature – but I desire that you understand the necessity of healing the mental body in order to reach true health alignment. In relation to the mental body, we are used to thinking about our conscious mind, but not necessarily the unconscious one. Hence, the unconscious is largely overlooked. But mental healing is the deepest level where we can seek assistance in healing from others – this can be profoundly impactful to create big positive shifts in our lives. In the next chapter, we talk about spiritual health. While others may assist us on this journey, you will see that this is much more of a personal experience. We can be encouraged, but spirituality is largely experienced on our own.

When we heal on the mental level, it affects every level below. This is why the therapies described above address physical, energetic, emotional and mental symptoms, sometimes all at once... Wow, powerful stuff! Mental healing creates profound, lasting change in every aspect of our reality.

ELEVEN

Fifth Level: Spiritual Body

"We are not human beings having a spiritual experience. We are
spiritual beings having a human experience."
~ *Pierre Teilhard de Chardin*

This is an excerpt from a writer, patient and friend, Johanna Olson,
on her spiritual journey:

*"For years I thought that moments of anxiety were evidence of my
ungodliness. Each moment of a sped up heart, a sweaty palm, or a racing
train of thought was accelerated by the fear that its presence meant a great
darkness in me.*

*In Philippians, Paul says "be anxious for nothing." Initially, I read this as a
reprimanding command against anxiety. A finger waving in front of my
nose, telling me that I have not trusted God in the way I should have. But in a
moment of divine grace and revelation, God revealed to me that his words are
actually ones of comfort. Instead of reprimanding readers for feeling moments
of anxiety, he is meeting them in the midst of their struggle [and] telling them
that they need not stay in a place of anxiety; he made the way out. His perfect
love expels all fear. His strength works best in our weakness.*

But still. Those monsters poke their heads out from under the bed. As much as you know that God brings peace, sometimes it seems hard to shake the gripping moments of anxiety, let alone the existence of anxious moments. When your mind is consumed by anxious thoughts, it seems antithetical and unauthentic to all of a sudden start telling yourself positive/faith-filled things. We're like hamsters committed to running our wheels to the end of their course, neglecting to step back and realize that the wheel never ends. How do we learn to walk in the things of God when it all seems theoretical, but we need practical?

Even though we invite God to dwell inside of us, to consume us, to make His words our words and His hands, our hands... we will never fully become God because we are us. We are the human conduits of the spirit of God. We are human beings in which the spirit of God dwells. But we're still human beings. And our relationship with God is still a relationship. It's part him and part us. Part of [the] journey is learning to be transformed by the God in us and then allowing that God in us to seep out of us and transform the world around us.

There will always be taunting voices and seductive lies that want to redefine who we are; people and situations that want to tell us that the worst is about to happen and we are not brave enough to handle it. This is why God reminds us that we have been given a "spirit not of fear but of power and love and self-control" (2 Timothy 1:7). It's like he's telling us he understands how we feel, but is reaffirming that fear is not from him.

Despite the circumstances that surround us, the Bible indicates that we are a mine of supernatural power. We need not go any further than our own spirits to stir up words of faith and encouragement in order to expel the surrounding atmosphere of anxiety.

I've realized that the important thing is not getting it right every time. The important thing is journeying closer to the equator of God within my spirit. To not fight my internal battles with topical ointments, but to allow the spirit of God to bubble up inside of me and transform my position against the world around me. I know God's not thinking less of me because of anxious moments, but I also know that he loves me enough to have already offered to carry the weights that are too big for me to carry."[88]

Whatever your faith or religion, I chose to include this story in this chapter because it shows how the essence of healing on this level is required to be internal. Spiritual health must come from within, from your divine experience with your Creator. Becoming healthy in this area is not something that a healer or practitioner can do *for* you. In fact, if they claim they can, I would suggest you turn and run. Spirituality is a personal journey and practice, and although others, such as pastors, priests, monks, gurus, theologians, rabbis or other spiritual leaders may support and guide you, it is solely up to you to embrace this journey.

What is Spiritual Health?

The spiritual level of healing brings a sense of oneness, bliss and the experience of God (or to Christians, the Holy Spirit). You access your higher levels of consciousness, also known as the seventh chakra, to develop the spiritual realms of purpose and connection.

This is the experience of spiritual awareness and health: a space where we feel deeply understood and feel unconditionally loved; a space where there are no limitations or judgments; a place where we belong; an area of utter completion where all sickness is repelled. The pure love of God is the only kind of love that can heal us in this way. And it doesn't come in pill form. We internally strive for this love in all of our relationships, despite our human imperfection.

Religions of the world have become a part of society's spiritual journey – a place for learning and connection to God that helps you become the best version of yourself, as divine creation intended. Unfortunately, history hasn't always painted the best picture of organized religion. Man's desire for personal power has sometimes created manipulation, confusion, misrepresentation, and even worse, death and destruction, in the name of religion. However, as God is omniscient and omnipotent, his design and purpose are not restricted to the confines to which humans through history have dictated.

No matter how you define your connection to a higher power, spirituality affects your health through your own development of a sense of spiritual coherence and unity with God. As described by Oprah Winfrey, "Spirituality is the measure of how willing we are to allow Grace – some power greater than ourselves – to enter our lives and guide us along our way." Religion can be a part of your spiritual journey, but it is not a requirement to create a space of healing. In this book I am not talking about your salvation, rather how spirituality can be developed to bring us wellness.

The Spiritual Journey

When we strive for spiritual awakening, we open the truth of fully knowing ourselves. This awakening is the framework to which your spirit knows the truth – *you are already created perfectly in God's image.* Meaning in your quest for spiritual healing you are not *becoming* spiritually healthy, you already *are.* It is a matter of peeling away the layers of obstacles to that actuality; you are spiritually complete exactly as you are. There is nothing to be added or taken away, just known and experienced.

Your perspectives, biases and stories have distorted this real truth. We feel that we are somehow flawed or broken, but you are already whole, complete and connected. What if you are exactly who you are supposed to be? And in fact, if you do not allow yourself to be as you truly are, you are depriving someone else of the authentic version of you. Your authentic self is deeply and divinely connected to your place on this earth. You're not supposed to be the famous person in the magazine that society tells you that you should look and act like – or the couple down the street with the flashy car, big house and "perfect life" – you're supposed to be you, the one and only you.

You have been given a divine spiritual purpose, being on this earth as you are, right now, in this moment of time, in the exact space that you were born, with the family that you came from. How do you find your purpose? It is wrapped up in the things you are gifted at, the things you enjoy and the ways in which you contribute to this world. Yup, that's right. This human experience of life is not about what you can get out of this world, but rather what your spirit can give it, your contribution. That internal fulfillment you get when you do something good for the world around you, with no material reward. Ask yourself:

1. How do I want to leave this earth?
2. What legacy will I leave for the next generation?
3. Will I continue a cycle of pain and hurt, or recognize my perfect spirit within, which is dying to be acknowledged and felt?

Pure love and acceptance; this is the goal. Only then can we transform and know that nothing in this physical existence is permanent. Your actual physical existence is merely the only limitation to the capacity you have on this earth, which is why we have talked so much about the necessity to keep all levels of health optimal. Remember our horse drawn carriage analogy? The purpose of the whole thing – the physical body, the energetic body, the emotional body and the mental body – is to facilitate the existence of your spiritual body on this earth. To transport you, the spiritual passenger of the carriage, down your path of destiny.

When we recognize our path is about (1) finding spaces and moments where we can have pure spiritual awareness and oneness, (2) feeling fulfillment from our personal contributions, and (3) recognizing that our divine nature is of wholeness and wellness, we can transform our health on all levels. We can then see that spiritual wholeness is not just an achievement or something we must come to deserve. Unconditional love for yourself and by God means there's nothing you can or cannot do to deserve supernatural transformations in your life. So whatever you have done or did not do, know that there are no special requirements to receive love and spiritual connection.

Everyone has a story. In this story you may feel there is a reason why you're not enough in some capacity or another. Or perhaps some past experience or wrongdoing made you feel unworthy to have complete power over your life, with freedom of love and acceptance for yourself. But I will tell you, that's a lie.

Maybe you've been manipulated into doing something that brings guilt and shame. Maybe you've been abused or raped and feel broken inside. Maybe you survived something that was traumatic or difficult that left you feeling resentful, fearful, guilty, angry or shameful. Maybe you hurt someone physically, mentally or emotionally... and maybe you even did it on purpose. Maybe the very people who were supposed to love you didn't, and in turn you feel unlovable. There are any number of experiences that can bring feelings of unworthiness. But know this, your spirit is not about other people, others' beliefs, others' actions or others' judgments. No one on this earth has authority over your spirit, and anyone telling you otherwise is creating lies that mask this truth. Your spirit is whole and you can heal your spiritual connection if you choose. Choose to let go of the self-punishment, self-judgment, and faulty-stories, and follow that internal God given conscience.

You do not need to live in the disconnection and lies. These perceived weaknesses or flaws have put on masks of undeserving. Yet, this feeling of brokenness is really the perfect space for God to work. As it says in the Bible, "My grace is sufficient for you, for my power is made perfect in weakness!" (2 Corinthians 12:9 NIV). What?! You don't have to be perfect to receive perfect healing love? Nope. The healing that can come from that understanding and realization can be instantaneous, complete and positively impact your health on every single level! Forgiveness and love is accessible to each and every one of you, but only if you make that choice.

Mosaic Books

411 Bernard Ave, Kelowna, BC
250-763-4418 or 800-663-1225
GST#115387854
orders@mosaicbooks.ca

Open 7 days a week, 363 days a year
mosaicbooks.ca

Fri Jul14-23 9:27am
Acct: 114767 Inv: I37318 P 00
Neil Webber

Qty	Price Disc	Total Tax

9781999404109 Courageous Cure,The: Under
| 1 | 31.50 | 31.50 a |

| | Subtotal | 31.50 |
| | a GST   5% | 1.58 |

| Items | 1 Total | 33.08 |
| (194/01901Z) | MCard | 33.08 |

======== Frequent Buyer Status =========
Credit earned with this purchase $ 1.26
Total credit on your account $ 5.56
Minimum required for redemption $ 10.00
===

-------------Card transaction ----------------
(retain for your records)
Resp. : APPROVAL
Type : CREDIT SALE MCARD
Acct : ***********3194   CAD $33.08
OurRef: 02280676
PmtRef: 528241764
MID   : ********703 TID: *****41A
Auth : 01901Z   PNRef: 528241764
Entry : INSERT PinVerified
AID   : PC Mastercard A0000000041010

CUSTOMER COPY

--------- Exchange Policy ----------
Full refunds for all product are
valid for 30 days after purchase.
Exchanges are valid for 60 days aft
er purchase. Products must be in
new condition and original
packaging.

Spontaneous Healing Miracles

Spiritual healing is witnessed in the miraculous. You can also call it divine intervention, spontaneous healing or spiritual alignment. I experienced divine healing myself in my central nervous system. It's not because I deserved to be healed – because I worked hard enough, said enough prayers, was disciplined enough in my eating, helped enough people and so on. It was only because I trusted and believed, with all of my heart, that I would be healed. I had faith and conviction in the healing, without attachment to how it would come about. I stepped into that faith with the intended action to do everything in my power to create healing, and I left what was out of my control to God, which means I had to let go of the idea that I was going to have it all under control and figured out. Sometimes we don't get what we want when we pray or ask for it, but we do get what we need, we just may not know it yet. The waiting process is a reminder to remember that life is a journey, not a destination.

Miracles are not fantasy, they happen to all of us and are all around us – the problem is, we don't always recognize them. Sometimes they are small – for example, somehow arriving at an appointment on time despite heavy traffic, or finding money come your way when you needed it and didn't know how you would make it work. Sometimes miracles are bigger – like "randomly" meeting the exact type of person you were requiring in your life at that moment, or somehow recovering from an illness or accident beyond what "the doctors" expected. This is spiritual synchronicity. I'm sure if you start to look at your own life, you can start to see those blessings too.

The trust or faith that you can create a desired change or outcome, outside your own realm of possibility, transpires on the spiritual level. This is "out of our control." No action you could have done, or strong will you had, could have solely created the change. Some may call it coincidence, but I challenge the way that we try to rationalize the unexplainable. To normalize and simplify the miraculous mysteries of our world and our nature, is to lose their awe and power. We see evidence of this idea even in the realm of science, where they are seeking what they call the "God particle" – the link between science and spirituality.

We are both the conscious and unconscious creators of our lives. There is a spiritual connectedness between all living beings on this earth. Many cultural groups throughout history, like many indigenous peoples, strongly recognized interconnectedness not only between humans, but also with all plants and animals, providing great respect and care for all living things. This connectedness breeds life. The First Nations cultures in Canada are rooted in balance and harmony with the earth. We could all learn from these traditions – if we do not show care to the earth, but rather allow destruction, it will also not care and nourish us. We need the earth, not only for food and shelter, but also for health and wellness. Nature can be one of the most amazing places to create spiritual connection. It helps us recognize our humanness and demonstrates how we impact and connect to everything around us.

THERAPIES FOR THE SPIRITUAL BODY:

Again, recognize that this is a personal spiritual experience. However, classical ways which people will connect and experience their individual spiritual oneness with God are prayer, inspirational music, being in nature, transcendental meditation, chanting, art, dancing or reading a spiritual text, like the Bible or Koran. For you, there may be something else where you feel spiritually connected.

The personal nature of spiritual healing means that what works for one person doesn't necessarily work for another. For example, the ways that I most strongly feel my spiritual connection to God are through song and through nature. I feel so united to everything around me when I'm adrift in the sounds and smells of God's wilderness.

Most likely you've experienced this connection before without realizing it. Maybe you were dancing, and felt connected to everything around you. You felt complete, loved, content and free. You felt joyous or even overwhelmed. I can spontaneously weep when I feel this Holy Spirit or spiritual oneness with God, even though there is no emotion of sadness.

The more we seek that connection, with universal truths and healing, the more alignment we have throughout our bodies. We can find this alignment by being in the present moment, and focusing on the now. In the here and now is where we can feel true peace, freedom, inspiration and awareness. When we uncover the ability to show complete forgiveness, love and acceptance towards ourselves, all the lies and illusions that have kept us from our truth will begin to dissolve. We also find the power to forgive others who have wronged us because we know the divine truth, *their* lies are what's keeping them from feeling and showing love. For a person to inflict pain on another, their hurts are ever more present inside and their spirit is masked in the falsehood of being unworthy of love.

As with all forms of healing, this journey to love and forgiveness will not likely happen all at once. This is a *process*, not a one-time deal. It may take a lifetime to reveal all the spiritual untruths that have been keeping you from recognizing your true peaceful, vibrant, powerful self. But trust that where you are today, is exactly where you are meant to be. That every experience has brought you to the awareness and opportunities you presently have. You don't have a crystal ball to the future, so you need to trust the process and let things reveal in their divine timing. Sometimes we also have to let go of the fear of being well, just as much as the fear of being sick. There may be significant change or responsibility in your life once you become well, are you ready for reality? Perhaps that's actually one of your most important blocks to overcome in order to become well.

No matter where you are in the voyage to wellness, if you don't feel like you have overcome the health challenges in your life, then know that the journey is not yet over. "For I know the plans I have for you," declares the LORD, "plans to prosper you and not to harm you, plans to give you hope and a future" (Jeremiah 29:11). The best is yet to come, this is the promise! You and all of humanity have the *choice* of whether to receive that promise… to step into your courageous cure.

Summary

As is written by Danny Silk in *Keep Your Love On*, "Shalom is a powerful Hebrew word that encompasses the flourishing of divine order, divine health and divine prosperity in your life. It means that every part of your life – body, soul, spirit, relationships, dreams and work – is being nourished and is growing and thriving. Shalom is literally the reality of God's kingdom of righteousness, peace and joy being expressed in your life."[89] This quote eloquently shows how, when we accept ourselves fully – through connecting to our spiritual nature and feeling its impervious love – we can recognize nothing is impossible. We can overcome. We can heal. We can expect miracles. We can find peace and joy and freedom, no matter the circumstances. As our spirit is everlasting, so too is God's love.

Conclusion

"I am not a product of my circumstances.
I am a product of my decisions."
~ *Stephen Covey*

When I decided to write this book, I knew if I could help just one person understand their own power to take control of their life and their health, it would be worth it. I pray that at this point, you have gained that understanding. Your body is not out to get you. You didn't do something to deserve suffering. Your body is not your worst enemy.

Your body is your personal vehicle to experience this physical life. Each symptom you experience is a particular message your body is trying to communicate. It's there to get your attention. To tell you that something needs to come into alignment, be balanced or become synchronized. That there is a conflict between one level in the body and another. Perhaps we are doing something that deep down inside we don't want to be doing. Or perhaps we are not doing something we wish we were doing… following a dream, speaking our desires and needs, changing a relationship, and so on. It's a judgement of our circumstances that creates this conflict. Thus, the body is unconsciously trying to resolve the conflict for you.

For example, various symptoms can be connected to a deeper meaning in the body:

- *Skin is related to sensation and touch. Hence, wanting a loving touch, but feeling undeserving perhaps due to a past trauma might manifest as a skin condition. Conversely, experiencing an unwanted touch can likewise create symptoms in the skin?*
- *Hypothyroid symptoms could be connected to feeling like life is moving faster than you want it to, so in turn your body slows down the only thing it can, you?*
- *Feeling like you have a hard time letting something go could in turn develop constipation?*
- *Believing that you are not moving forward in life and feeling pain in the knees?*
- *Feeling held back in life and experiencing hip pain?*
- *Believing that you are not supported by someone in the way you want, and in turn developing back pain?*
- *Avoiding or dissociating from a situation or circumstance and creating numbness in the body?*

I could go on, but the common thread is that each area has a specific meaning and message. You need only think of the function of that area in the body and it will give you a clue. Symptoms do not happen by chance. The body doesn't make mistakes. We were created with accuracy and precision. And the body is designed to heal. It's doing the best job it can.

This particular point of time in your life is a product of all the decisions, consciously and unconsciously, that you've made along the way. The accumulation of decisions and actions, or inactions, has led you to this very moment. This realization is not a message of condemnation. You did not intentionally create all these symptoms you are suffering from. Yes, you are the director of your current reality, but you are also the instrument of your revolution and change. Therefore, this realization will actually bring you freedom, because you now can make a different choice at any point in your health journey. You can optimize your circumstances to the best capacity possible.

This understanding is a gift from your awareness. There is no turning back now, because now you know. You can grab hold of your courage, and be the creator of your optimal, individual, best version of you. Choose to be well, strong, energetic, healed and vibrant. When you take ownership of that choice, then and only then will you understand your full capability to create your destiny. This requires accountability for your actions, responsibility for your behaviours, and acknowledgement of where you need help.

Illness is a messenger to help you see this truth. A truth that is accessible to any human being. It's your birthright to be healthy. Instead of looking for a label to justify your existence or sickness, understand that you are already complete, you are already healed. When you simply make that decision, then every action and behaviour has to fall in line with that. What you have struggled with, going on willpower alone, will suddenly become easy. From quitting smoking, to changing your diet, to incorporating exercise, to changing your attitude, you will feel empowered to accomplish it. You have no idea the power that you have within you, if you just make the choice to step into it. Own it. Will it be instantaneous? Maybe, maybe not. Maybe it's just the start of a journey towards freedom and health. To work towards being pain free, worry free or fearless.

We are interconnected with everything around us, and when we step into our decision to be healthy, everything around us will support us in that path. The opportunities will show up, the people will arrive, the circumstances will begin to change. The universe is there for us to shape into our chosen reality. This is synchronicity. Wouldn't you rather create what you want consciously, rather than what you don't want, unconsciously? You have that power.

This thing holding you back, this pain, this suffering, whatever root cause we are talking about – it doesn't need to be permanent. It does not define you – you define you. What do you want to be defined by: anger, frustration, pain, fear, blame, resentment, bitterness or shame, or strength, resilience, courage, kindness, freedom, love, joy, passion or hope? This symptom or limitation you are dealing with has a purpose in your life – to show you something, to reveal a truth, to create an opportunity of understanding. You can find peace in all things.

Everyone's journey is different. Everyone's path to understanding is different. The outcome may not always look the way you want it to, as the physical body does have its limitations, we are not immortal. Regardless, the lessons for growth and purpose are always there. Sometimes to receive them, we have to let go of the need to control the result and just embark on the journey. There is no way to know at which point your physical capacity is reached – and I also don't believe anyone can tell you that. I do believe if we commit to the journey and seek our deepest healing, we can leave that restoration to the inner wisdom of the body.

When you dig into the root causes of disease, and in turn, figure out how you need to heal, you are changing the course of your future. As a free gift to you with the purchase of this book, I'd like to help you walk through your own personal action plan workbook that you can access through www.thecourageouscure.com. Enter the password: *createyourcure*. Together, we will make a plan on how to start making changes today.

When we release ourselves to this adventure, and let go of our need for the healing to look a certain way, we can then discover the true nature of our health journey. Disease is not your true form – it is not how you were created or a definition of who you are.

It's time to be the enlightened author of your life.

If you enjoyed this book and would like to share you comments with others, please leave a review at amazon.com, amazon.ca or google reviews.

You can also follow Dr. Berg on all of her social media channels @dralanaberg on Facebook, Instagram, Youtube, and Twitter.

Stay connected on her website at dralanaberg.com for updates, blogs, and courses offered.

References

References:

Chapter 1: Genetics

[1] Lipton, B. (2005). *The Biology of Belief: Unleashing the Power of Consciousness, Matter, & Miracles,* Authors Pub Corp.

Chapter 2: Nutrient Deficiencies

[2] Ledowsky, Caroline. (2015). "Vitamin B12 – The Reference Range Level is Set Too Low." *MTHFR Support.* Retrieved from:
https://www.mthfrsupport.com.au/vitamin-b12-reference-range-level-set-low/

[3] Smith, D. (2011). "Do we need to reconsider the desirable blood level of vitamin B12?" *Journal of Internal Medicine.* November.

[4] Davis, D.R., Epp, M.D., Hugh D. Riordan, H.D. (2013). "Changes in USDA Food Composition Data for 43 Garden Crops, 1950 to 1999." *Journal of the American College of Nutrition.* Vol. 23, No. 6669-682.

[5] Thomas, D.E. (2007). The Mineral Depletion of Foods Available to Us as a Nation (1940–2002) - A Review of the 6th Edition of MCance and Widdowson. *Literature Review in Nutrition and Health (Berkhamsted, Hertfordshire).* July. 19(1-2):21-55

[6] Picard, A. (2018). Today's fruits, vegetables lack yesterday's nutrition. *Globe and Mail.* April. Retrieved from
https://www.theglobeandmail.com/life/todays-fruits-vegetables-lack-yesterdays-nutrition/article4137315/

[7] Picard, A. (2018). *Today's fruits, vegetables lack yesterday's nutrition. Globe and Mail.* April. Retrieved from
https://www.theglobeandmail.com/life/todays-fruits-vegetables-lack-yesterdays-nutrition/article4137315/

[8] Loss, G. et al. (2011). "The protective effect of farm milk consumption on childhood asthma and atopy: The GABRIELA study." *Journal of Allergy and Clinical Immunology,* 128 (4), 766-773.

[9] Baxter-Jones, A., Faulkner, R., Forwood, M., Mirwald, R. and Bailey, D. (2011) "Bone mineral accrual from 8 to 30 years of age: An estimation of peak bone mass." *Journal of Bone and Mineral Research.* Retrieved from
https://onlinelibrary.wiley.com/doi/abs/10.1002/jbmr.412

Chapter 3: Toxicity

[10] Exposures Add Up - Survey Results (2004). *Environmental Working Group.* Retrieved from https://www.ewg.org/skindeep/2004/06/15/exposures-add-up-survey-results/#.WzFZalVKivE

[11] *National Toxicology Program* (2018). January 15. Retrieved from
https://ntp.niehs.nih.gov/about/

[12] Exposures Add Up - Survey Results (2004). *Environmental Working Group.*
Retrieved from https://www.ewg.org/skindeep/2004/06/15/exposures-add-up-
survey-results/#.WzFZalVKivE

[13] Finamore, A., Roselli, M., Britti, S., Monastra, G., Ambra, R., & Mengheri, E.
(2008). "Intestinal and peripheral immune response to MON810 maize ingestion in
weaning and old mice." *Journal of Agriculture and Food Chemistry.* 56 (23), pp
11533–11539

[14] Pusztai, A. (2001). "Genetically Modified Foods: Are They a Risk to
Human/Animal Health?" *ActionBioScience.org, American Institute of Biological
Sciences.* Retrieved from
http://www.globalmagazine.info/sites/default/files/PDF/pusztai-gm-foods-risk-
human-animal-health-2001.pdf

[15] Kokkonen, J., Arvonen, M., Va¨ha¨salo, P., & Karttunen, T. J. (2007). "Intestinal
immune activation in juvenile idiopathic arthritis and connective tissue disease."
Scandinavian Journal of Rheumatology. 36, 386-389.

[16] Vendomois, J. & Roullier, F. (2009). "The Comparison of The Effects of 3 GM
Corn Varieties on Mammilian Health." *International Journal of Biological Sciences.*
5(7), 706-729.

[17] World Centric: UN Food and Agriculture Association (2018). January 15.
Retrieved from http://worldcentric.org/conscious-living/social-and-economic-
injustice

[18] Seralini G. et al. (2014). Republished: "Long term toxicity of Roundup herbicide
and Roundup-tolerant genetically modified maize." *Environmental Sciences Europe.*
26,14.

[19] Toxin Nation. (2018). *Environmental Defence.* January. Toronto. Retrieved from
http://www.environmentaldefence.ca/toxicnation/home.php

[20] Government of Canada (2015). *Chemicals Management Plan: Progress Report,*
Fall Issue. Retrieved from http://www.ec.gc.ca/ese-
ees/default.asp?lang=En&n=B6D66F41-1

[21] Muir, T. & Zegarac, M. (2001). "Societal Costs of Exposure to Toxic Substances:
Economic and Health Costs of Four Case Studies That Are Candidates for
Environmental Causation." *Environmental Health Perspectives.* 109, 885-903.

[22] *United States Environmental Protection Agency* (2018, January 15). Retrieved
from https://www.epa.gov/indoor-air-quality-iaq/volatile-organic-compounds-
impact-indoor-air-quality

[23] International Agency for Cancer Research (2015). IARC Monographs. *World Health Organization.* 112. Retrieved from https://www.iarc.fr/en/media-centre/iarcnews/pdf/MonographVolume112.pdf

[24] Benbrook, C. (2016). "Trends in glyphosate herbicide use in the United States and globally." *Environmental Sciences Europe.* 28, 3.

[25] Grandjean, P. & Landrigan, P. (2014). "Neurobehavioural effects of developmental toxicity." *The Lancet Neurology.* 13, 330-338.

[26] Spalding K.L, Arner E., Westermark P.O., Bernard S., Buchholz B.A., Bergmann O., Blomqvist L., Hoffstedt J., Näslund E., Britton T., et al.(2008). "Dynamics of fat cell turnover in humans." *Nature, International Journal of Science*; 453:783-7; PMID:18454136; Retrieved from http://dx.doi.org/10.1038/nature06902

[27] *Stats Canada* (2018). "Lead, mercury, and cadmium concentrations in Canadians, 2012 and 2013." January. Retrieved from https://www.statcan.gc.ca/pub/82-625-x/2015001/article/14209-eng.htm

[28] Kern, J. et al. (2016). "The relationship between mercury and autism: A comprehensive review and discussion." *Journal of Trace Elements and Biology.* 37, 8-24.

[29] Chen, P., Miah, M., & Aschner, M. (2016). Metals and Neurodegeneration. *PubMed Central.* Retrieved from https://www.ncbi.nlm.nih.gov/pmc/articles/PMC4798150/

[30] Rowley, B. & Monestier, M. (2005). "Mechanisms of heavy metal-induced autoimmunity." *Molecular Immunology.* 42(7), 833-838.

[31] Rana, S. (2014). "Perspectives in endocrine toxicity to heavy metals – a review." *Biological Trace Elements Research.* 160(1), 1-14.

[32] *The Immunization Advisory Committee* (2018). Efficacy and Effectiveness. January. Retrieved from http://www.immune.org.nz/vaccines/efficiency-effectiveness

[33] *Institute of Medicine (U.S.) Immunization Safety Review Committee* (2018). Immunization safety review: multiple immunizations and immune dysfunction. January. Retrieved from https://www.ncbi.nlm.nih.gov/books/NBK220493/

[34] Institute of Medicine. (2013). *The Childhood Immunization Schedule and Safety: Stakeholder Concerns, Scientific Evidence, and Future Studies.* Washington, DC: The National Academies Press. https://doi.org/10.17226/13563.

[35] Mawson, A., et al. (2017). "Pilot Comparative Study on the health of vaccinated and unvaccinated 6- to 12-year-old US children." *Journal of Translation Science.* 3(3), 1-12.

[36] Obukhanych, T. (2012). *Vaccine Illusion: How vaccination compromises our natural immunity and what we can do to regain our health.* GreenMedInfo LLC.

Chapter 4: Chronic Infections

[37] Cassel, G. (1998). "Infectious Causes of Chronic Inflammatory Diseases and Cancer." *CDC Emerging Infectious Diseases Journal:* September, 4 (3).

[38] Romagnani, S. (1996). "Th1 and TH2 in Human Disease." *Clinical Immunology and Immunopathology:* September, Volume 8 (3): 225-235.

[39] Singh, V. et al. (1999). "The Paradigm of Th1 and TH2 cytokines, It's relevance in Auto-immunity and Allergy." *Immunologic Research:* December V 20, (3): 147–161.

[40] Huggins, H.A., Levy, T.E. (1998). *Uninformed Consent: The Hidden Dangers in Dental Care.* Hampton Roads Publishing Company.

[41] Morsczeck, C. and Reichert, TE. (2018). "Dental stem cell in tooth regeneration and repair in the future." *Expert Opinion on Biological Therapy.* February;18 (2):187-196

[42] Segal, I. (2010). *The Secret Language of Your Body: The Essential Guide to Health and Wellness.* Beyond Words Publishing.

[43] Zangger, H. et al. (2013) "Detection of Leishmania RNA virus in Leishmania parasites." *PLOS Neglected Tropical Diseases.* 7(1)

[44] Cohen, S. et al. (2003). "Emotional Style and Susceptibility to the Common Cold." *Psychosomatic Medicine.* July, 65 (4): 652-657.

[45] Segal, I. (2010). *The Secret Language of Your Body: The Essential Guide to Health and Wellness.* Beyond Words Publishing.

[46] Lipton, B. (2005). *The Biology of Belief: Unleashing the Power of Consciousness, Matter, & Miracles,* Authors Pub Corp.

[47] Cohen, S. Pressman, D. (2006). "Positive Affect and Health." *Sage Journals.* June 1, 15 (3): 122-125. Retrieved from http://journals.sagepub.com/doi/pdf/10.1111/j.0963-7214.2006.00420.x

Chapter 5: EMF – Electromagnetic Frequencies

[48] Radiation risk from everyday devices assessed, (Published 17 Sep 2007 - Last modified 21 Jun 2016), *European Environment Agency.* Retrieved from https://www.eea.europa.eu/highlights/radiation-risk-from-everyday-devices-assessed

[49] *BioInitiatives Report* (2012). "A Rationale for Biologically-based Exposure Standards for Low-intensity Electromagnetic Radiation." Retrieved from http://www.bioinitiative.org

[50] McTaggart, L. (2008). *The Field: The Quest for the Secret Force of the Universe*. Harper Perennial.

[51] *BioInitiatives Report* (2012). "A Rationale for Biologically-based Exposure Standards for Low-intensity Electromagnetic Radiation." Retrieved from http://www.bioinitiative.org

[52] Suk, W. (2009). Environmental Factors in Cancer. *Meeting Summary of President's Cancer Panel*. Phoenix, Arizona.

[53] *BioInitiatives Report* (2007). "A Rationale for Biologically-based Exposure Standards for Low-intensity Electromagnetic Radiation." Retrieved from http://www.bioinitiative.org

[54] Deshmukh PS, Megha K, Banerjee BD, Ahmed RS, Chandna S, Abegaonkar MP, Tripathi AK. (2013). "Detection of Low Level Microwave Radiation Induced Deoxyribonucleic Acid Damage Vis-à-vis Genotoxicity in Brain of Fischer Rats." *International Journal of Toxicology*. 20(1):19-24.

[55] Redmayne, M., Smith, E., and Abramson, MJ. (2013). "The relationship between adolescents' well-being and their wireless phone use: a cross-sectional study." *Environmental Health*, 12(1):90.

[56] Regel, SJ, Tinguely, G, Schuderer, J, Adam, M, Kuster, N, Landolt, HP, Achermann, P., (2007). "Pulsed radio-frequency electromagnetic fields: dose-dependent effects on sleep, the sleep EEG and cognitive performance." *Journal of Sleep Research.* 16(3):253-258.

[57] Gye, Myung Chan and Park, Chan Jin., (2012). "Effect of electromagnetic field exposure on the reproductive system." *Clinical and Experimental Reproduction*. March, 39(1):1–9.

[58] Yang, X.S., He, G.L., Hao, Y.T., Xiao, Y., Chen, C.H., Zhang, G.B., Yu, Z.P. (2012). "Exposure to 2.45 GHz electromagnetic fields elicits an HSP-related stress response in rat hippocampus." *Brain Research Bulletin*. 88(4):371-378.

[59] Aldad, T.S., Gan, G., Gao, X.B., Taylor, H.S. (2012). "Fetal radiofrequency radiation exposure from 800-1900 MHz-rated cellular telephones affects neurodevelopment and behavior in mice." *International Journal of Scientific Reports.* 2:312.

[60] Sokolovic, D., Djordjevic, B., Kocic, G., Babovic, P., Ristic, G., Stanojkovic, Z., Sokolovic, D.M., Veljkovic, A., Jankovic A., Radovanovic, Z. (2012). "The effect of melatonin on body mass and behaviour of rats during an exposure to microwave radiation from mobile phone." *The International Journal Bratislava Medical Journal.* 113(5):265-269.

[61] Akbari, A., Jelodar, G., Nazifi, S. (2014). "Vitamin C protects rat cerebellum and encephalon from oxidative stress following exposure to radiofrequency wave

generated by a BTS antenna model." *Toxicology Mechanisms and Methods.* 24(5):347-352.

[62] Carpenter, D. (2010). "Environmental Fields and Cancer: The Cost of Doing Nothing." *Reviews on Environmental Health.* January 25 (1): 75-79.

[63] Naziroğlu, M, Gümral, N. (2009). "Modulator effects of L-carnitine and selenium on wireless devices (2.45 GHz)-induced oxidative stress and electroencephalography records in brain of rat." *International Journal of Radiation Biology.* 85(8):680-689.

[64] Schoeni, A, Roser, K, Röösli, M. (2015). "Memory performance, wireless communication and exposure to radiofrequency electromagnetic fields: A prospective cohort study in adolescents." *Environment International.* 85:343-351.

Chapter 6: Stress and Trauma

[65] Selye, H. (1936). "A Syndrome produced by diverse nocuous agents." *Nature, International Journal of Science.* 138: 32.

[66] Sapolsky, R.M. (2004). *Why Zebras Don't Get Ulcers: The Acclaimed Guide to Stress, Stress-Related Diseases, and Coping.* Holt Paperbacks; 3rd edition.

[67] Salleh, M.R. (2008). "Life Event, Stress and Illness." *Malaysian Journal of Medical Sciences;* October, 15(4): 9–18. Retrieved from https://www.ncbi.nlm.nih.gov/pmc/articles/PMC3341916/

[68] Feletti, V. et al. (1998). "Relationship of Childhood Abuse and Household Dysfunction to Many of the Leading Causes of Death in Adults." *American Journal of Preventive Medicine.* Volume 14, pages 245–258.

[69] Gratrix, N. (2016). "The 7 Steps to Healing Childhood Emotional Trauma and Building Resilience." February. Retrieved from https://www.nikigratrix.com/how-to-build-resilience-and-resolve-emotional-trauma/.

Part 2 Introduction

[70] Soler, J. (2015). *Adventure of the Soul: The Art of Listening to Life & the Art of Alignment.* Infinity Publishing.

Chapter 7: 1st Level of healing – The Physical Body

[71] D'Adamo, P.J., Whitney,C (1997). *Eat Right 4 Your Type (Revised and Updated): The Individualized Blood Type Diet Solution.* Penguin Publishing Group.

[72] Metchnikoff, E. (1908). *The Prolongation of Life: Optimistic Studies.* English translation: Mitchell, P.C., GP Putnam's Sons, New York.

[73] Utz, J. (2016). "The water in you." *U.S. Geological Survey.* Retrieved from https://water.usgs.gov/edu/propertyyou.html

[74] The Safe Mercury Amalgam Removal Technique (SMART) (2016). *International Academy of Oral Medicine and Toxicology.* Retrieved from https://iaomt.org/resources/safe-removal-amalgam-fillings/

[75] Dirty Dozen. (2018). *EWG's 2018 Shopper's Guide to Pesticides in Produce™.* ewg.org. Retrieved from: https://www.ewg.org/foodnews/dirty-dozen.php

[76] Pharmaceuticals in drinking-water. (2012). *World Health Organization.* http://www.who.int/water_sanitation_health/publications/2012/pharmaceuticals/en/

Chapter 8: 2nd Level of healing - The Energetic Body

[77] Payán, Fischer, Cardozo, Andrade, Pinilla (2017). Proceedings from *the International Neural Therapy Conference.* Ottawa, Canada.

[78] *BioInitiatives Report.* "A Rationale for Biologically-based Exposure Standards for Low-intensity Electromagnetic Radiation." Retrieved from http://www.bioinitiative.org

Chapter 9: 3rd Level of Healing - The Emotional Body

[79] Vishen Lakhiani (2017). *Breaking All the Brules.* Impact Theory. April. Retrieved from www.youtube.com/watch?v=BvpAeRGnkJ4

Chapter 10: 4th Level of Healing – The Mental Body

[80] The Conscious, Subconscious, And Unconscious Mind – How Does It All Work? (2014). *The Mind Unleashed.* March. Retrieved from https://themindunleashed.com/2014/03/conscious-subconscious-unconscious-mind-work.html

[81] Brown, Brené (2015). *Rising Strong.* Random House Publishing Group.

[82] Maruna, S., and Copes, H. (2005). "What Have We Learned from Five Decades of Neutralization Research?" *Crime and Justice*, Vol. 32, pp. 221-320

[83] Myss, C. (1998). *Why People Don't Heal And How They Can.* Harmony.

[84] Brown, Brené (2015). *Rising Strong.* Random House Publishing Group.

[85] McCraty, R., Atkinson, M., and Bradley, R. (2004). "Electrophysiological Evidence of Intuition: Part 2. A System-Wide Process?" *The Journal of Alternative and Complementary Medicine.* Vol 10, Num. 2: pp. 325-336.

[86] What is Intuition(2012). *Math of Heart Math*, October 8. Retrieved from: https://www.heart.math.org/articles-of-the-heart/the-math-of-heartmath/what-is-intuition/

[87] Singer, M.A. (2007). *The Untethered Soul: The Journey Beyond Yourself.* New Harbinger Publications/ Noetic Books.

Chapter 11: Level 5 – Spiritual Body

[88] Olson, Johanna. Kelowna, British Columbia, Canada

[89] Silk, D. (2015). *Keep Your Love On: Connection Communication And Boundaries.* Loving On Purpose Ministries.

About the Author

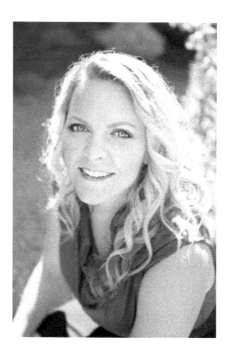

Dr. Alana Berg, originally from Alberta, Canada, discovered at a very young age her desire to help people. This led her to a path of pre-medical training at the University of Alberta, and ultimately to the profession of Naturopathic Medicine, graduating from the Canadian College of Naturopathic Medicine in 2005. She began a full-time practice in 2006, and embarked on developing and honing her professional skills. She has achieved certification by the College of Naturopathic Physicians of British Columbia in: chelation, acupuncture, IV therapy, pharmacology, and ozone. As well, she has trained in neural therapy, trigger point injections, Bodytalk therapy, Neuropsychokine-siology, and several other courses along the way. Other expertise has been gained directly from working with other doctors and practitioners from the United States, across Western Canada, Mexico and Spain, in order to fully dive into the healing arts. She has worked in integrative practices over the years, and currently practices in her clinic Axiom Health, in Kelowna BC, where she has resided since 2006.

She has a general family practice, with a special interest in Lyme disease and chronic infections, detoxification and environmental medicine, digestive conditions, auto-immune diseases, men's and women's health, and stress management.

She has also always been very excited about education; and she has been heard as an expert on 1150 AM radio, seen on CHBC TV news health tips, and has presented at many forums and public groups on various topics. Her deep passion for healthy living and desire to teach and empower others, has given her a great commitment and dedication to her field. Furthermore, with her own health journey in healing Multiple Sclerosis, she deepened her understanding of health and healing. All of this encouraged her to now shift gears to take this passion to the next level and create this book.

She enjoys her off time with her beautiful family, husband Robertson, and daughters Myla and Haylee. They love the outdoors and exploring their beautiful Okanagan home; skiing, hiking, and camping regularly. Travel is a passion, and they regularly incorporate it as much as they can. Both she and her husband have a heart for Africa, having supported, created, and participated in mission trips to the region. Ten percent of all the proceeds from this book will be going to charities that she supports.

For more information:
www.dralanaberg.com

CPSIA information can be obtained
at www.ICGtesting.com
Printed in the USA
LVHW070525290623
751055LV00004B/499